Enhancing
Medication Adherence:
The Public Health Dilemma

Enhancing Medication Adherence: The Public Health Dilemma

Editor
Hayden B Bosworth, PhD
Duke University Medical Center
Durham VA Medical Center
Durham, NC

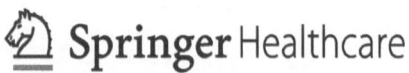

Published by Springer Healthcare Ltd, 236 Gray's Inn Road, London, WC1X 8HB, UK.

www.springerhealthcare.com

British Library Cataloguing-in-Publication Data.

A catalogue record for this book is available from the British Library.

ISBN 978-1-908517-47-0

Although every effort has been made to ensure that drug doses and other information are presented accurately in this publication, the ultimate responsibility rests with the prescribing physician. Neither the publisher nor the authors can be held responsible for errors or for any consequences arising from the use of the information contained herein. Any product mentioned in this publication should be used in accordance with the prescribing information prepared by the manufacturers. No claims or endorsements are made for any drug or compound at present under clinical investigation.

Project editor: Tess Salazar
Designer: Joe Harvey
Artworker: Sissan Mollerfors
Production: Marina Maher
Printed in Great Britain by Latimer Trend

Contents

Author biography

Hayden B Bosworth, PhD, a health services researcher, focuses on patient and organization level factors to improve treatment adherence. He is the associate director of the Center for Health Services Research in Primary Care and Career Award scientist at the Durham Veterans Affairs Medical Center (VAMC). He is a research professor in the Department of Medicine, Division of General Internal Medicine, research professor in the Department of Psychiatry and Behavioral Sciences, research professor in the School of Nursing at Duke University Medical Center, and adjunct professor in the Department of Health Policy and Administration in the School of Public Health at the University of North Carolina at Chapel Hill. He is also a senior fellow at the Center for Aging and Human Development and a senior fellow at the Center for Health Policy at Duke University. Dr Bosworth was awarded an Established Investigator award from the American Heart Association to further develop interventions to improve health behaviors and treatment adherence related to hypertension and other chronic diseases. Dr Bosworth has published over 180 articles and 3 books that have examined the self-management and treatment adherence among individuals with chronic diseases. He is a fellow of the American Psychological Association Division 20 (Adult Development and Aging and Division 38 Health Psychology), Gerontological Society of America, and the Society of Behavioral Medicine. He has received prior funding from a number of government sources (eg, National Institutes of Health, Veterans Affairs) and foundations (eg, American Heart Association, Robert Wood Johnson Foundation) to carry out three overarching areas of research: 1) clinical research that provides knowledge for improving patients' treatment adherence and self-management in chronic care; 2) translation research to improve access to quality of care; and 3) eliminate healthcare disparities.

In terms of treatment adherence in chronic care, Dr Bosworth has expertise developing interventions to improve health behaviors related to chronic diseases, including coronary artery disease, diabetes, and depression, and has been developing and implementing tailored patient interventions to reduce the burden of these chronic diseases for the last 15 years. His research contributions to the field of health psychology and behavioral medicine, specifically health behaviors, memory and cognitive ability, social support, depression, and risk perception, all factors associated with treatment adherence, are all reflected in his on-going work. This work has resulted in significant improvements in outcomes and testing of methods of revising healthcare systems to provide efficacious care in a cost effective way to as many people as possible.

Abbreviations

AAFP	American Academy of Family Physicians
AAP	American Academy of Pediatrics
ACP	American College of Physicians
AOA	American Osteopathic Association
CMS	Centers for Medicare & Medicaid Services
CI	confidence interval
EHR	electronic health record
Health IT	health information technology
HHS	United States Department of Health and Human Services
MEMS	Medication Event Monitoring System™
MMAS	Morisky Medication Adherence Scale
PCMH	patient-centered medical home model
RCT	randomized controlled trial
SDM	shared-decision making
WHO	World Health Organization

Abbreviations

PART ONE

Understanding medication nonadherence

Chapter 1

Defining medication nonadherence

Introduction

Medications are the primary tools used to prevent and effectively manage chronic illness; however, despite their importance and known benefit, appropriate medication use remains a challenge for both patients and providers. Patients frequently do not adhere to essential medications, resulting in poor clinical outcomes, increased cost of care, and deleterious consequences for workforce productivity and overall public health [1]. An estimated half of the 3.2 billion annual prescriptions dispensed in the USA are not taken as prescribed [2]. Numerous studies have shown that patients with chronic conditions adhere to only 50–60% of medications as prescribed, despite evidence that medical therapy can reduce mortality and improve quality of life [3–8]. Adherence to prescription medication has been labeled as our "other drug problem" [9], an "epidemic" [10], and a "worldwide problem of striking magnitude" [1].

Adherence to prescribed medications is directly associated with improved clinical outcomes, higher quality of life, and lower healthcare costs across many chronic conditions [1–8]. An estimated 125,000 deaths per year in the USA are due to medication nonadherence [11], and between 33% and 69% of medication-related hospital admissions in the USA are due to poor adherence [2]. However, the true rate of nonadherence may be higher as patients with a history of nonadherence are likely to be underrepresented in clinical trials outcomes research [1]. The lost opportunity for effective therapies to improve health is staggering.

H. B. Bosworth, *Enhancing Medication Adherence: The Public Health Dilemma*, DOI: 10.1007/978-1-908517-66-1_1,
© Springer Healthcare 2012

For example, cardiovascular medications alone are responsible for half of the 50% reduction in mortality from coronary heart disease over the past 20 years [12]; yet actual achievement of these cardiovascular benefits is lost due to high rates of nonadherence in real-world settings.

At its most obvious, poor adherence worsens morbidity and increases mortality [1], which directly harms patients and indirectly impacts their family and friends. Poor adherence also exacerbates physical and psychiatric disabilities [13], affecting family, work, and other social responsibilities, including parenting and wage earning. Medication nonadherence channels limited health funds in directions that could be used better elsewhere [13], and contributes to healthcare provider over utility. Medication nonadherence may also lead to society-wide outbreaks of diseases that could have been eliminated by population-wide vaccination. For some conditions (eg, a few psychiatric and neurologic disorders), it may even imperil the public by directly or indirectly leading to increased crime and unnecessary accidents. Improving medication adherence may be one of the most effective ways to address chronic medical conditions [1,12].

There is also growing evidence that improved medication adherence may not only improve clinical outcomes but also reduce medical costs [13,14]. For example, in the USA, higher adherence to renin–angiotensin–aldosterone system inhibitors and statins by Medicare beneficiaries with diabetes resulted in a lower cumulative Medicare spending over 3 years [15]. On the other hand, nonadherence increases healthcare costs for payers and employers [12,16] and contributes to inferior beneficiary outcomes. For pharmaceutical companies and pharmacies, nonadherence has been associated with significant revenue loss.

Definition and measurement of medication nonadherence

Medication adherence refers to the extent to which patients follow provider recommendations about day-to-day treatment with respect to the timing, dosage, and frequency of their prescribed medications [1,17,18]. It may be defined as "the extent to which a patient acts in accordance with the prescribed interval and dose of a dosing regimen" [17].

Medication persistence refers to the duration of medication-taking, and is defined as "the duration of time from initiation to discontinuation of therapy" [17]. The International Society for Pharmacoeconomics and Outcomes Research considers "adherence" and "compliance" to be synonyms [17]. The World Health Organization (WHO) recognizes two distinct categories of nonadherence – preventable (eg, patient forgets, misunderstands) and nonpreventable (eg, life-threatening side effects) – and recommends tailored treatment interventions for the former [1].

Medication adherence may also be defined as the extent to which people follow the instructions they are given for prescribed treatments [19]; it involves consumer choice and is intended to be nonjudgmental, unlike compliance, which reinforces patient passivity and blame. On the other hand, concordance refers to an emerging consultative and consensual partnership between the consumer and their prescriber [19]. Medication nonadherence includes delaying prescription fills, failing to fill prescriptions, cutting dosages, and reducing the frequency of administration.

Medication nonadherence can be further defined as primary or secondary nonadherence. Primary nonadherence (not initially filling the prescription written) for example, has been shown to lead to a significant increase in 1-year mortality after hospitalization for myocardial infarction [20], and it is estimated that up to 20% of myocardial infarction patients do not fill a new prescription [20,21]; primary nonadherence appears to vary by therapeutic class [22]. Secondary nonadherence (failure to follow the instructions or to refill the prescription) has been shown to increase mortality, hospitalizations, and costs [23]. Primary nonadherence has received less attention because of the challenges of identifying individuals given a medication prescription but failing to fill it.

Medication nonadherence has also been conceptualized as having two additional components [24]:

1. A purposeful decision-making process wherein patients intentionally choose to stop taking their medication due to beliefs or perceptions about medication.
2. An unintentional, random departure from taking medication due to factors such as forgetfulness, interruption of daily routines, inability to access medications, or lack of reminders.

Once a patient obtains a medication, the two most common nonadherent behaviors include omitting one or more doses or taking a medication at the wrong time [25]. Consumption of extra doses is less common [26,27]. Comprehension of the prescribed regimen is the first step in successfully complying with the regimen. Studies have reported that one-fifth to one-half of elderly patients have difficulty understanding or lack knowledge about their medication regimen [28,29]. Patients may confuse the role and use of their medications, particularly with more complicated regimens. For example, patients with moderate-to-severe asthma are prescribed two forms of medication, a daily anti-inflammatory medication and a "use as needed" bronchodilator to administer when they have symptoms. When patients are interviewed about their understanding of these two medications, there are often gaps in their knowledge about which of these medications is prescribed to treat the symptoms of an asthma attack [30].

> **❝** *A written medication schedule or figure with instructions can often enhance adherence [31].* **❞**

Rudd has termed the behavior of inconsistent adherers as "partial compliance" [25]. Electronic medication monitors indicate that about 50–60% of patients achieve near-optimal or excellent adherence, and 5–10% of patients display low levels of adherence, with long periods of taking no medications at all. Partial compliers, who represent the remaining 30–45% of patients, display highly variable adherence, with day-to-day and week-to-week inconsistencies [26]. For example, for some patients weekday adherence presents no problem, but weekends or holidays disrupt medication routines. Partial compliers appear to understand their regimen and the need for pill taking, yet they skip doses or sometimes take "drug holidays" for up to weeks at a time. This is particularly the case among patients with HIV/AIDS, where interruptions of highly-active antiretroviral therapy (HAART) have been suggested to help manage the toxic effects of therapy; however, recent research has found that these drug holidays are associated with greater progression of disease and do not confer immunologic or virologic benefits to patients [32].

While partial adherence is intentional in some patients, it may be unintentional in others. Forgetting to take a medication is the most common cause of underdosing. Cognition and memory plays an important role in adherence and control [33–35], particularly among older adults [36]. In data from the Framingham Heart Study, a strong-graded relation between cognitive performance, including memory, and the probability of having stopped antihypertensive medication use, was reported [37]; those in the lowest 10th percentile of education-adjusted cognitive performance were over three times as likely to have stopped treatment than those in the normal performance group [38].

Unintentional partial adherence often occurs in scheduling when to take a medication. When patients skip or are off-schedule with doses, for example, they often skip or are off-schedule with all medications taken at that time [38]. For instance, if a patient sleeps through a morning dose of medication(s) or is late taking an evening dose because of being delayed at work, all medications taken at that time are missed or delayed. Partial adherence or nonadherence may also be affected by such factors as using more than one pharmacy, seeing a number of different physicians, confusion about the regimen, inaccurately labeled containers, and, among older adults and those with problems with arthritis, the inability to open childproof containers [39]. Each of these behaviors must be considered in formulating strategies to enhance medication treatment adherence for patients [40].

> **"** *It is important to point out that what seems like a straightforward behavior, such as taking a pill on a regular schedule, is actually a complex endeavor.* **"**

Successful pharmacologic treatment of any medical condition requires patient adherence in a multistep pathway [2] that includes:
1. Keeping a scheduled appointment with a provider.
2. Accepting a prescription for a medication.
3. Filling the prescription at a pharmacy.
4. Taking the medication as prescribed.
5. Maintaining an adequate supply of the medication by refilling the prescription in a timely manner.
6. Returning to the provider for ongoing monitoring.

Chapter 2

Causes of medication nonadherence

" *Between 100 and 250 factors have been observed to be associated with medication nonadherence [41,42], thus making the importance of tailoring management to individuals' needs and using a multifaceted approach very apparent [43].* "

Adherence research has unsuccessfully tried to find clear correlations between fixed patient characteristics, such as age, gender, or education, and adherent or nonadherent behavior [44,45]. However, when moving beyond these sociodemographic variables, modifiable patient characteristics, such as behavior and attitudes, have been shown to be barriers to medication adherence. For example, forgetfulness, fear of undesired side effects, reservations toward drug taking, and insufficient educational information and understanding about drug therapy or drug holidays have been found to be related to medication nonadherence [46].

A report by the WHO addressed the general importance of improving adherence to long-term medical treatments [1]. The WHO report concluded that adherence is the result of a complex interaction of the social environment, patients, and healthcare professionals. It has been shown that low adherence to long-term treatment often occurs when the treatment is complex or when the disease is asymptomatic (such as hypertension). Previous studies have reported that poor adherence to too many drugs is due to patient perception that the disease is not significant, adverse drug effects, lack of treatment effectiveness, and the patient's

H. B. Bosworth, *Enhancing Medication Adherence: The Public Health Dilemma*, DOI: 10.1007/978-1-908517-66-1_2, © Springer Healthcare 2012

poor or incomplete knowledge of the disease [47]. Known barriers can be characterized in at least three [42] ways:

1. Health literacy barriers related to not knowing what to do and why.
2. Behavioral barriers that address not having the skills necessary to accomplish medication management in the context of everyday life.
3. System or administrative barriers related to access and fragmentation of care.

Thus, the most effective interventions use a combination of approaches and address literacy, behavior, and organizational issues. System or administrative factors are derived from a patient's inability to afford or difficulty in affording their medication and may include, for example, lack of adequate healthcare coverage, unemployment, retirement, and indigence.

Patient-level factors related to medication nonadherence

The most common reasons given by patients for not taking their medications are forgetfulness (30%), other priorities (16%), deciding to omit a dose (11%), lack of information (9%), and emotional reasons (7%); 27% of patients give no reason [48]. Factors that are associated negatively with adherence include increased complexity or duration of a medication regimen, side effects, very old age, extreme poverty, social isolation, and psychiatric diagnoses, especially paranoia [49]; a study on adherence in HIV-positive individuals, which included these patient-level factors, found that older HIV-positive patients with neurocognitive impairments or drug problems were at an increased risk of suboptimal medication adherence when compared to their younger counterparts (Figure 1) [50]. The risk of nonadherence is especially high when multiple predisposing factors converge, such as cognitive impairment and the use of numerous medications for multiple chronic conditions in the elderly.

In general, important predictors of adherence in single conditions include the use of simple and short regimens, particular classes of medications favored by consumers, and a high severity of disease and symptom score [12]. Older adults' and consumers' beliefs that therapy will help are additional predictors of adherence [12]. Key reasons for nonadherence include adverse effects or other problems with medications, such as poor

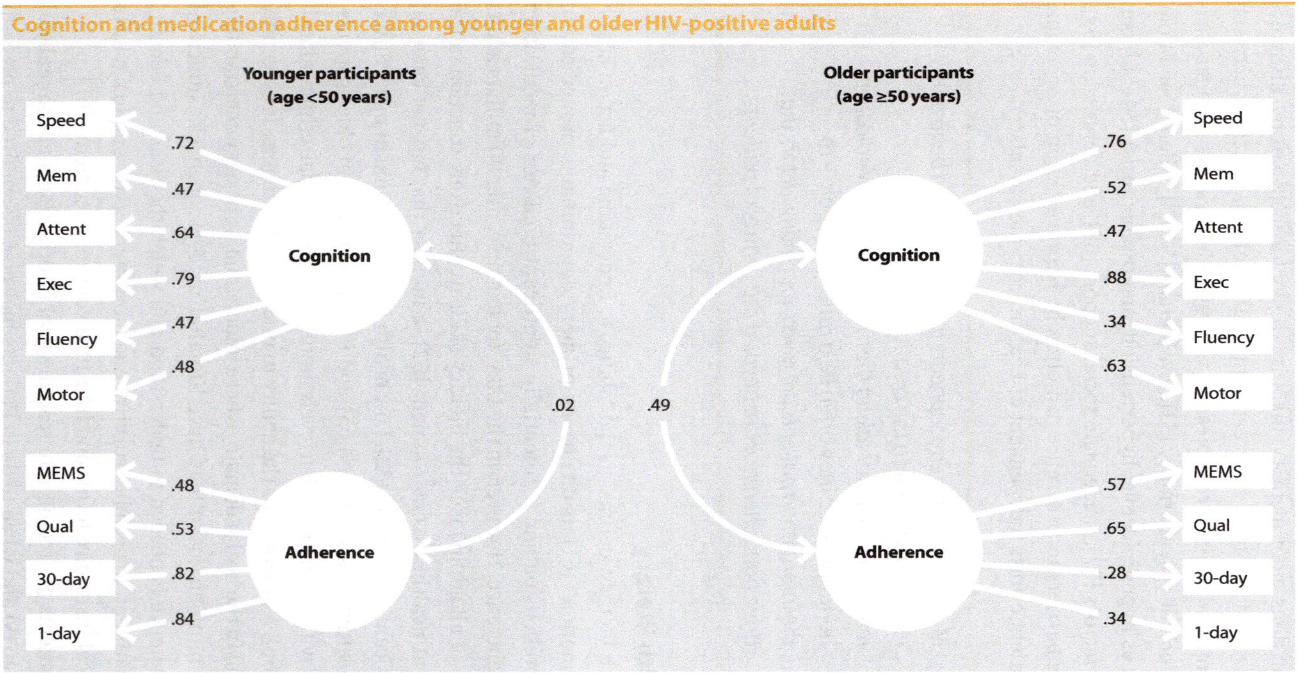

Figure 1 Cognition and medication adherence among younger and older HIV-positive adults. 1-day, 1-day self-report; 30-day, 30-day self-report; Attent, attention; Exec, executive; Mem, memory; Qual, qualitative self-report. Standardized values shown. Reproduced with permission from Gorman AA et al [50].

instructions, poor memory, inability to pay for medications, disagreement about the need for treatment, and weak relationships between patients and healthcare professionals [19]. Other reasons for nonadherence include polypharmacy [51], low literacy [52,53], "silent" conditions (such as hyperlipidemia, hypertension, and osteoporosis) [54–56], cultural factors [57], inadequate social support [58], and depression [59]. These barriers to adherence can often be improved upon or overcome by patient efforts independent of healthcare professionals.

> *Medication adherence appears to be a patterned behavior established through the creation of a routine and a reminder system for taking the medication [60]. Medication nonadherence may often be a rational response to the information patients are given, and many factors that drive nonadherence are beyond the control of patients.*

Health literacy

Health literacy, defined as the "ability to understand and act on health information" [61], is one of the primary determinants of medication comprehension and a potentially significant predictor of medication nonadherence. However, in the USA, for example, over 90 million adults (39% of all adults) lack the literacy skills to effectively function in the current healthcare environment [62], a number that has not changed significantly over time [63]. Low health literacy is found in many different healthcare settings [64,65] and is most common in older patients, those with lower education levels, immigrants, and racial/ethnic minorities [66]. Numeracy, or the ability to understand numbers, is especially critical in the health domain, where understanding or not understanding what numbers mean may have life-altering consequences. Numerical competence is needed to understand and weigh the risks and benefits of treatment, to decipher survival and mortality curves, and to navigate medical insurance forms and informed consent documents [67].

Patients are required to read medical information and comprehend what to do and when to do it. Patients may also be required to perform numerical tasks, including calculating the number of tablets for a single dose of medicine. They are expected to monitor themselves for both beneficial and adverse effects of their medications, know what to do if they miss a dose of medication, and master when, if, and how to obtain refills [68]. Chronic illnesses often require following an intensive and complex medical regimen (eg, medications, daily monitoring, routine physician visits, and tests), such that the adverse consequences of low health literacy may be particularly pronounced and thus require serious consideration [69]. Methods for screening for health literacy include a number of measures as well as asking patients if they have a problem understanding written health materials (see Figure 2) [70,71].

Self-efficacy

The key to self-management of chronic conditions is self-efficacy, or the confidence to carry out behaviors necessary to reach a goal identified by the patient [72]. Self-efficacy has been reported to improve medication adherence in studies employing survey and/or focus-group methods [73]. Studies using interview techniques have reported numerous medication compliance problems in people with multiple chronic conditions [74–76]. For example, medications for one condition can negatively affect another condition, and managing schedules that require medications at different times as well as pill burden can be major deterrents to achieving adherence [77]. A synthesis of qualitative studies of why there is resistance to taking medications showed that people were concerned about taking medications for long-term chronic conditions

Patients' understanding of their medication and adherence	
Medication knowledge	**Patients answering correctly (%)**
Dose	65.6
Frequency	49.2
Indication	19.7
Monitoring method	**Patient adherence (%)**
MEMS measurement	30.0
Prescription refill assessment	38.0

Figure 2 Patients' understanding of their medication and adherence. MEMS, Medication Events Monitoring System. Reproduced with permission from Hauptman [71].

because of potential adverse effects. As a result, they "actively resisted" taking their medications rather than being forgetful, as cited by other researchers [77].

Physician-level factors related to medication nonadherence

Perhaps because patients take the medications, most of the attention on medication nonadherence focuses on the patients themselves; however, Tarn et al suggest that physician behaviors may critically contribute to medication nonadherence [78]. Not only is the ability of physicians to recognize nonadherence poor, they often lack adequate training to alleviate problems. Tarn et al documented major deficits in the information and education that physicians give to patients when prescribing new medications [78]. Physicians frequently omitted critical information, such as the name of the medication, purpose of the medication, duration of treatment, dosing schedule, and associated adverse effects of new medications. The data showed that in over 65% of all cases, at least one critical piece of information was not provided [78].

Barriers to adherence may also be related to poor interactions and/or communication between patients, healthcare providers, and the healthcare system. Traditionally, physicians and designated healthcare workers have played a key role in achieving adherence by providing patients with the rationale for treatment and involving family and caregivers whenever possible; however, it is time and resource intensive for providers to assess and influence adherence alone on a timely and ongoing basis. There remains an unmet need for reliable and broadly utilizable ways to accurately assess and manage a patient's medication adherence.

> *An ideal system for improving adherence would not only engage the patients themselves, but also leverage their selected healthcare providers, caregivers, and communal support network. The system would also allow a secure exchange of reliable and robust information among patients and clinical decision and support systems [79].*

Healthcare system-level factors related to medication nonadherence

For many patients, the cost of medication directly affects their level of medication adherence. In the USA, for example, the coverage gap in Part D for patients on Medicare may be a financial challenge, particularly for expensive medications; however, sometimes generic alternatives provided at lower cost can provide a solution. Additionally, several studies have shown a strong and consistent relationship between copayments and medication adherence [80–83]. A substantial portion of medication nonadherence is driven by out-of-pocket costs of multiple medications [84–86]. Patients with chronic illness are likely to skip or discontinue their medications in response to copayment increases [81,87]. Unfortunately, those with multiple chronic conditions (and presumably using more medications) are more susceptible to cost-related nonadherence [84], which may exacerbate chronic conditions, generate adverse health events, and increase healthcare use [88,89].

Payers and healthcare plans could turn this information to an advantage. Payers could selectively reduce or eliminate copayments for highly beneficial medications for some patient subgroups, such as statins in patients with heart disease or diabetes or blood pressure-lowering medications for those with hypertension. This has led to a movement, known as "value-based insurance design," to reduce copayments for the most effective, high-value medications [90,91]. Observational studies have found that reducing copayments for highly effective chronic therapies can substantially improve adherence [91,92]. Moreover, studies suggest that adherence improves when physicians prescribe generic or lower-cost medications [93].

Others have posited that simply reducing copayments may not be sufficient, and have proposed that providing financial rewards for better adherence may be an even more effective mechanism for promoting behavior change. Volpp et al found a significant impact from financial incentives to improve smoking cessation rates [94], as well as for promoting weight loss [95]. While physician pay-for-performance has received substantial attention in the medical literature, patient pay-for-performance is a concept that needs further research in order to understand its long-term effectiveness and cost-effectiveness.

Moving toward adherence-dependent quality and performance measures

Consistent with current emphases on quality, access, and equity of care [96], the literature focuses on performance measures in which medication adherence contributes to quality scorecards, including mortality, more intermediate treatment targets such as blood pressure and lipid control, and decreased symptom-associated readmissions [97–101]. The link between medication adherence and treatment targets is robust, although practical approaches that help patients improve medication adherence are lacking. For this reason, the WHO has distinguished between modifiable and nonmodifiable risk determinants. In a clinical setting, nonmodifiable factors might serve as "flags" to alert providers to communicate carefully with patients, whereas modifiable factors might serve to trigger specific interventions for patient-associated adherence problems [139].

Chapter 3

Methods for determining medication adherence

The methods available for measuring adherence can be broken down into indirect and direct methods of measurement. Each method has associated advantages and disadvantages, and no method is currently considered to be the gold standard [102,103].

Indirect methods for determining medication adherence

Indirect methods of measuring adherence include asking the patient about how easy it is to take prescribed medications, assessing clinical response, performing pill counts, ascertaining rates of refilling prescriptions, collecting patient questionnaires, using electronic medication monitors, measuring physiologic markers, asking the patient to keep a medication diary, and assessing children's adherence with the help of a caregiver, school nurse, or teacher. Questioning the patient (or using a questionnaire), using patient diaries, and assessing clinical responses are all relatively easy methods to use, but questioning the patient can be susceptible to misrepresentation and tends to result in the healthcare provider overestimating adherence.

Measurement models have sought to replace fundamentally categorical considerations (eg, "Did the patient take her meds? Yes or no?") with more continuous ones [104]. Poor adherence, for instance, is likely to vary over time. For example, many patients do not quit medication altogether; medication adherence waxes and wanes and is rarely an always or never

H. B. Bosworth, *Enhancing Medication Adherence: The Public Health Dilemma*, DOI: 10.1007/978-1-908517-66-1_3, © Springer Healthcare 2012

proposition. Variability of administration may be explained by symptoms, reinforcement of illness behaviors, costs and availability of services, and cultural relevance of treatments. These questions are variable from patient to patient and over time in terms of the direction of effects, and are influenced by treatment outcomes and quality of life.

Clinicians must frequently rely on their own judgment, but unfortunately this often is no better than chance-accuracy in predicting patient adherence [105]. Thus, alternative methods for assessing medication adherence are needed.

Medication adherence is commonly measured in one of three ways:
1. Patient self-report.
2. Pharmacy refill records.
3. Use of electronic equipment, such as the Medication Event Monitoring System (MEMS™) Caps (AARDEX Group, Sion, Switzerland).

These measures are limited by the degree of separation between the time and place of the measurement process and actual behavior. For example, self-report measures of medication adherence rely on patients' perceptions of their behavior and are subject to recall and reporting bias [106,107]. Prescription refill records provide the prescribed medication quantity, but do not verify actual dosing or taking of medications [106,107]. The approach using an electronic device to capture a dosing event and time is often considered the reference standard for measuring adherence, but these devices may not always precisely capture when or how much of the medication was ingested [106,108].

Data suggest that these various measures of medication adherence may be assessing different but related concepts that may influence medication adherence. In one study reviewing a sample of primary care patients with hypertension, agreement between medication acquisition as assessed by a centralized pill refill and a commonly used 4-item measure of self-reported medication adherence (Morisky self-report measure), indicated a significant but poor agreement ($\kappa=0.19$, $P<0.001$) [109]; however, in another study, both pill acquisition (undersupply and oversupply) and self-reported nonadherence were independently associated with a decreased likelihood of blood pressure control, after adjusting for each other and patient factors [110]. Thus, measures of pill refill (ie, medication acquisition) and self-reported adherence appear to provide distinct, complementary information about patients' medication-taking behaviors.

In a recent meta-analysis examining the associations between MEMS and self-reported questionnaires, the pooled correlation coefficient for 11 studies was 0.45 (95% confidence interval [CI], 0.34–0.56), indicating that there is at least a moderate association between MEMS and self-reported measures of medication adherence [111].

A clinically based cut-off point of 80% is commonly used to differentiate between medication adherence and nonadherence, although skepticism exists about such cut-off points because there are very few medications for which a clinically relevant cut-off point has been empirically studied [112]. In addition, for some medications, such as HAART, adherence levels need to exceed 80%. In studies of adherence in patients with heart failure or hypertension, the commonly used cut-off point of 80% demonstrated a reasonable balance between sensitivity and specificity [113]. In addition, all measures provided similar estimates of overall adherence, although refill and electronic measures were in highest agreement [113].

Unlike other methods of measuring adherence, self-report is simple and economically feasible and has the added advantage of soliciting information regarding situational factors that interfere with medication adherence, for instance forgetfulness and adverse effects [114–116]. As such, self-report is a widely adopted method for assessing medication adherence; however, patients tend to overestimate their medication adherence [117], and unless a patient is not responding to therapy, it may be extremely difficult to identify poor medication adherence.

" A key, nonjudgmental, validated question is, "Have you missed any pills in the past week?" and any indication of having missed one or more pills may signal a problem with low adherence [118]. "

Compared to pill counts as the reference standard, asking nonresponders about their medication adherence using this single question will detect 55% of those with less than complete adherence, with a specificity of

87% (likelihood ratio +4.3 [95% CI, 3.1–6.1]; likelihood ratio –0.51 [95% CI, 0.44–0.58]) [105].

Patients generally want to please their physicians and will often say what they think their doctor wants to hear. It can be reassuring to the patient when the physician tells them, "I know it must be difficult to take all your medications regularly. How often do you miss taking them?" This approach makes most patients feel comfortable in telling the truth and facilitates the identification of poor adherence. A patient who admits to poor adherence is generally being candid [119]. Patients should also be asked whether they are having any side effects from their medications, whether they know why they are taking their medications, and what the benefits of taking them are, since the responses to these questions can often expose poor adherence to a regimen [109].

Another practical method for identifying poor medication adherence involves awareness of timing. Patients' adherence to treatment is greatest in the period 5 days prior to and 5 days after their appointment with their healthcare provider and usually tapers off significantly within 30 days – the so-called "white-coat adherence" effect [2].

While self-reported measures of medication adherence are commonly used, they are subject to social desirability bias, recall bias, and response bias. Self-reported measures have also been criticized for poor reliability and distributional properties (eg, restricted range and skewness). Self-reported medication nonadherence rates are estimated to be 10–20% lower than the rates obtained with other methods [120,121]. Consequently, there have been concerns raised about the use of self-report measures [122,123].

66 *Physicians should have a heightened awareness of the possibility of poor adherence, but even patients in whom these indicators are absent can miss taking medications as prescribed. Thus, poor adherence should always be considered when a patient's condition is not responding to therapy.* 99

Adherence scales

The Morisky scale is a commonly used, validated, 4-item self-reported adherence measure that has been shown to be predictive of medication adherence [109,124]. Morisky et al updated the original measure so that it now includes 8 items – the Morisky Medication Adherence Scale (MMAS) [125]. Each of the 8 items evaluates a specific medication-taking behavior rather than determinants of adherence behavior, and thus better captures the barriers surrounding adherence behavior. The MMAS has been shown to have higher reliability compared to the original 4-item scale (α=0.83 versus 0.61) [125]. MMAS scores can range from 0 to 8 and have been trichotomized previously into three levels of adherence [125] to facilitate use in clinical practice:

1. High adherence (MMAS score of 8).
2. Medium adherence (MMAS scores of 6–<8).
3. Low adherence (MMAS scores of <6).

In the case of hypertension, one study has revealed that the new scale is significantly ($P<0.05$) associated with blood pressure control with 67.2% of low adherers having uncontrolled blood pressure versus 55.2% and 43.3% of medium and high adherers, respectively [125]. Concordance between MMAS and continuous single-interval medication availability, medication possession ratio, and continuous multiple-interval medication gaps was greater than or equal to 75% [125].

Another brief self-report measure of medication adherence is the Adherence Estimator [126]. Patients can be placed into one of three segments based on the total score: low-, medium-, and high-risk for non-adherence. Sensitivity was 88% for the nonadherers, such that 88% of patients identified as being at a medium- or high-risk for nonadherence are accurately classified by the Adherence Estimator [126].

Pharmacy refills and pill counts

Clinicians may conduct pill counts or review pharmacy records, if available. A substantial portion of the adherence literature is based on estimates obtained from pharmacy-claims databases, in part because such databases are a relatively inexpensive and accessible tool for obtaining medication refill data across large populations. Pill refill has been suggested as an important quality measure. A recognized limitation to the use of pharmacy claims is that adherence can only be estimated for patients who have purchased the drug (ie, an insurance claim) [2,9].

Pharmacy refill records may provide a reliable and nonintrusive longitudinal measure of medication adherence; however, it is necessary that all patients obtain their medication from a centralized pharmacy, such as the US Department of Veterans Affairs or other integrated healthcare systems, in order to keep track of medication refills. Pill-refill records do not give any indication of when the medication was taken or whether it was thrown away, and thus may result in overestimation of adherence. In addition, this method of assessing medication adherence requires extensive data-tracking programs. Lastly, pill-refill measures typically exclude primary nonadherence (ie, not filling a prescription) and potentially may underestimate the true rate of medication adherence by up to 20% [20,21].

Another type of information uniquely provided by refill adherence measures relates to the identification of patients who accumulate excesses of prescribed medication, in addition to those with insufficient supplies for adherence. Oversupply of medication, or refilling medications more frequently than required for adherence, may be problematic if it reflects or leads to intentional or unintentional overuse of medication or sharing of medications with others. Even if patients do not consume or share excess medication, oversupply may reflect an inefficient use of healthcare resources (eg, stockpiling, frequent loss, and replacement of medications).

The few studies considering oversupply as a distinct phenomenon have linked oversupply to higher total healthcare costs and risk of hospitalization [127–129], although the reasons for these associations and whether they are causal are poorly understood. While these studies highlighted oversupply as common and potentially problematic, there is a current dearth of research describing characteristics of patients with oversupply [27,130].

Electronic measurement devices or microelectric event monitoring

Electronic monitors, including the MEMS Caps, consist of a microprocessor placed in a medication container with a switch that is activated by the interruption of an electrical current. When activated, the microprocessor records the date and time the bottle was opened. Several months of data can be stored on these units before they need to be downloaded onto a computer. These medication monitors can provide information on the pattern of drug intake, including the frequency and timing of medication dosing over a fairly extended period of time [131]. Measures of adherence computed using data obtained by MEMS Caps include:

1. MEMS adherence rate: the number of days on which a MEMS Caps was opened at least once divided by the number of days of monitoring by MEMS, then multiplied by 100. This reflects the percentage of days on which at least one dose was presumed to have been taken. If an individual does not open the pill bottle on a particular day, that day is coded as a nonadherence day.

2. The prescribed intervals method, which quantitates the fraction of doses taken at the prescribed dosing intervals. If the prescribed dosing frequency was 12 hours (for a twice-daily regimen), then a dosing event was considered adherent if it occurred within 10–14 hours of the previous dosing event. Prescribed intervals are calculated by the number of prescribed dosing intervals plus or minus 2 hours, divided by the total number of possible intervals [131].

Other electronic monitors can be used to assess medication adherence, including tablet-blister packs, pill rings, eyedrop solution bottles, and aerosol spray nebulizers. Variations on electronic monitors are also being developed. For example, there are devices that report medication patterns to a provider via telephone and modems, and related information can be used to reorder medications. Devices are also being tested that not only record when a medication cap is open, but can be programmed to inform the user through various methods (ie, noise or flashing light) that a medication dosage is due.

Electronic monitors are not widely available and are relatively expensive. Adherence assessment via electronic devices may produce "reactivity" (ie, the assessment activity itself tends to move the behavior in the socially desirable or therapeutic direction). Furthermore, electronic monitors preclude the use of a pillbox to organize the medication being monitored by the electronic cap, and some patients remove more than one dose per bottle opening to avoid carrying around the medication bottle when leaving home. In addition to inaccurate interpretations if multiple doses are removed at once, other limitations of this technology include the need for accompanying technology to interpret the readings of the computer chip and patient acceptance and accurate use of the computerized caps. Lastly, it is often challenging to monitor all medications that individuals are taking, yet assumptions can be made that adherence to one medication represents the potential adherence behavior for all other medications an individual is taking. These assumptions are not always valid and often adherence varies by medication. Such limitations may result in electronic monitoring underestimating a patient's actual adherence. Electronic monitored adherence rates consistently range between 10% and 20% lower than rates assessed by other methods, including self-reports [132] and pill counts [133].

Direct methods for determining medication adherence

Biological indices

Examples of direct methods of measures of medication adherence are directly observed therapy (ie, measurement of concentrations of a drug or its metabolite in blood or urine) and the detection or measurement in blood of a biologic marker added to the drug formulation. As a measure of medication adherence, these markers often are confounded with physiological differences among patients and with patient–drug inter-actions. For example, there are genetic differences in how individuals absorb, metabolize, and excrete drugs, and medication and urine levels can only be assessed during clinic visits. In addition, these assays can be expensive and the measurements can be misleading if the medication has a short serum half-life, as the patient may have taken their pills only just before the time of determination or may have misused just that dose.

In response to such limitations, biological tracer substances with minimal interindividual variation and long half-lives have been added to drugs [134,135]. For some medications, measuring biologic levels is a good and commonly used means of assessing adherence. For instance, the serum concentration of antiepileptic agents, such as phenytoin or valproic acid, will probably reflect adherence to regimens with these medications, and subtherapeutic levels will likely reflect poor adherence or suboptimal dose strengths. In summary, in a few cases, directly observed therapy may be needed and warrant the costs, but this is more likely to be the exception rather than the rule.

Supervised dosing

Supervised dosing has seldom been used to determine medication adherence, with the exception of antitubercular treatment [136,137], methadone for treatment of narcotic addiction, and monitoring of glycemic adherence in children with diabetes. Up to half the people with tuberculosis do not complete their treatment. A Cochrane review that compared policies of directly observed therapy for tuberculosis with self-treatment found that patients (n=1910) allocated to observed therapy had similar outcomes in relation to cure as did self-monitored patients (relative risk 1.06; 95% CI, 0.98–1.14) [137]. The obvious drawback of supervised dosing is its expense for the healthcare system and inconvenience for patients. It is usually only advocated in extreme cases where societal costs of non-adherence are obvious. While not reviewed here, there are also potential ethical issues related to supervised dosing.

PART TWO

Methods for addressing medication nonadherence

Chapter 4

Evaluating adherence-enhancing interventions

Brief summary of medication adherence studies and interventions

A number of systematic reviews evaluating adherence-enhancing interventions have been published in recent years. The Cochrane reviews of randomized controlled trials (RCTs) have assessed interventions for improving medication adherence for commonly occurring single-chronic conditions, such as diabetes, hypertension, and hyperlipidemia [54,55,138]. The reviews report methodologic problems and insufficient evidence to support adherence-enhancing strategies in these specific single conditions. Haynes et al identified effective ways to improve medication adherence for a variety of medical conditions in widely differing populations. Adherence to short-term drug treatment was improved by written information, personal phone calls, and counseling. For long-term treatments, no simple interventions and only some complex ones led to some improvement in health outcomes [12]. Schroeder and colleagues focused on medications for controlling blood pressure, and reported enhanced adherence by reducing the number of daily doses [54]. Patient support and education interventions that targeted practical medication management skills aimed at individuals' improved adherence to HAART [139]. Another review concluded that reminder packaging increased the proportion of people taking their medications, but the effect was not large [140]. Simple, low-cost interventions can enhance adherence to essential medications, may have significant public health

H. B. Bosworth, *Enhancing Medication Adherence: The Public Health Dilemma*, DOI: 10.1007/978-1-908517-66-1_4, © Springer Healthcare 2012

benefit, and may be a good investment to effectively address chronic medical conditions [1,141].

Medication adherence in the hospital

Poor medication adherence is more likely to occur in certain contexts. Medication problems are common in the transition period from hospital discharge to the outpatient setting, and often begin at the point of hospital discharge. For instance, nearly a quarter of patients who had an acute myocardial infarction were partially or completely nonadherent in filling prescriptions after discharge [20]. Of the patients who are initially adherent, up to 50% will discontinue antihypertensive medications within 6–12 months, and only about 40% continue statin medications for 2 years after hospitalization for acute coronary syndrome [142,143]. Makaryus et al found that less than 50% of patients were able to list all of their medications, and even fewer could recount the purpose of their medications at hospital discharge [144]. In addition, Coleman and colleagues found that medication discrepancies were common, occurring approximately 15% of the time, and patients with medication discrepancies were twice more likely to be rehospitalized within 30 days of discharge [145].

> *Methods shown to improve medication adherence are discharge medication counseling, positive interactions between clinician and patient, close follow-up with patients (1 to 2 weeks after discharge), low costs or copayments for prescription medications, and simplified drug regimens [12,20]. It may be helpful to initiate motivational strategies, including daily drug reminder charts, training on self-determination, reminders, social support, nurse telephone calls, family member support, and telephone-linked computer counseling [12].*

Medication adherence in the clinic

A crucial step in ensuring medication adherence is to determine whether the patient can communicate and process the information that the healthcare providers are sharing with them. If a healthcare provider is not able to effectively communicate with the patient, then monitoring prescription refills, counting pills, and involving friends and family members are of value when nonadherence is suspected [146,147].

> **"** *Asking patients to explain the reasons they are prescribed each medication may reveal their lack of understanding, which predicts a high likelihood of poor adherence. Providers should assess patients' daily schedules and medication-taking competency to develop and promote a medication routine.* **"**

The following factors potentially assist patients in maintaining good adherence by helping to minimize side effects or simplifying doses and regimens:

1. Electronic prescribing and use of shared electronic health records (EHRs) so that all healthcare providers are aware of prescribed medications.
2. Dosing aids.
3. Drugs, which are more acceptable to the patient and have reduced side effects.
4. Improved condition monitoring by doctors and patients.

Role of health information technology and electronic health records

> **"** *The ability to systematically collect, organize, access, analyze, and better understand health information using EHRs is expected to impact how medication adherence is monitored [148].* **"**

Electronic prescribing and integration of drug prescription information into the patient medical records provide important opportunities to measure and improve medication adherence. Health information technology (health IT) can help to connect patient, provider, pharmacy, and healthcare system data, and is already being used to generate important medication management and monitoring quality metrics. Led by the National Health and Human Services Office of Information

Technology, incentives to integrate health IT into physician practices with parameters that fulfill "meaningful use" criteria enables the integration of measurements of medication adherence as well as tools to improve adherence, which could be extremely important toward meeting the ultimate goal of improved medication adherence.

Electronic prescribing and the potential to use health IT offer significant opportunities to measure and improve medication adherence by capturing and providing notifications from the pharmacy to the prescriber when the prescription is, or is not, filled. When medication information is shared electronically, prescribers have access to information that allows them to assess a patient's medication regimen at the point of care and to identify nonadherence. Electronic systems may also be able to notify a prescriber or pharmacist about refills, which can help trigger an intervention to avoid a potential gap in medication use. Health information exchange can facilitate medication reconciliation by providing a means for healthcare providers to capture a patient's complete medication list. Other members of a healthcare team may also retrieve that information to reconcile medications across the care continuum, during transitions of care, hospital admissions, and hospital discharge.

In the USA, the Centers for Medicare & Medicaid Services (CMS) in the Department of Health and Human Services (HHS) provides incentives to encourage the "meaningful use" of certified EHR technology by eligible healthcare professionals and hospitals. In order to receive incentive payments, the CMS requires eligible professionals and hospitals to meet certain measures, some of which support improved medication adherence by using certified EHRs. The Office of the National Coordinator for Health IT has established standards and certification criteria for certified EHRs to enable professionals and hospitals to meet these measures [149].

Some of the measures and the related criteria for certified EHRs functionality support efforts to improve medication management and medication adherence. For example, meaningful-use Stage One criteria includes requirements to maintain active medication and allergy lists and to generate prescriptions electronically for a specified percentage of patients. Stage One also includes an option for providers to perform medication reconciliation for transitions of care. Additional meaningful-use criteria in Stage One promote consumer empowerment by giving patients access to their information, including discharge instructions and patient summaries. This could assist with medication adherence by providing information to patients to help them understand the prescribed medications and instructions for taking those medications [150].

Health IT has the potential to provide alerts and reminders to both healthcare providers and patients to support medication adherence. As more data become available about factors that improve the likelihood of non-adherence, EHR functionality could use predictive modeling to identify patients who are the least likely to comply with medication regimens and enable targeted intervention to improve compliance. While the evidence regarding the role of health IT in interventions to improve adherence is quite thin, studies evaluating the role of electronic reminders show promise.

Consumer eHealth tools, such as personal health records and mobile phone applications, are being used to empower patients to play a more active role in managing their medications. These tools may provide electronic reminders to patients, allow patients to track their adherence, and in some instances provide real-time information back to the provider for intervention and/or targeted follow-up.

" This interactive capability is important, since some literature suggests that patient engagement is associated with improved treatment adherence. "

Pharmaceutical packaging

Innovative pharmaceutical packaging has the potential to leverage the therapeutic benefit of self-administered drugs substantially by reducing nonadherence. For example, medication packaging that incorporates a simple day or date calendar feature can prompt the patient to maintain the prescribed dosing schedule. Calendar pill organizers are plastic trays or boxes with separate compartments labeled with the days of the week, which generally are filled by the patient from pharmacy-dispensed vials containing loose pills. Calendar blister packaging is a unit-of-use (generally 1 month) packaging in which each pill's blister is labeled with the day of the week or date of the month, providing a visual record of when the patient last took their medicine [151].

Planar medical packaging

Chapter 5

The role of healthcare providers in medication adherence

Who should provide medication adherence interventions?

> " While physician time and select-skill sets may be limited to support improved adherence overall, physician endorsement of medication adherence and processes is critical. "

Findings from a recent review suggest that adherence interventions using a team approach with nonphysician healthcare professionals are effective in improving cardiovascular medication [152]. This is particularly important considering the high cost of physician time as compared to some other healthcare professionals. There is also a growing body of literature supporting a team approach, whether nurse/physician [153] or pharmacist/physician [153,154], to improve medication adherence.

The increased interest in the patient-centered medical home (PCMH) model of healthcare delivery will provide further insight into the optimal team to address medication adherence. Beginning in the 1980s, mostly in the pediatric sector, it was recognized by some that a physician-centric orientation was misplaced and interfered with the optimal care of chronically ill children. This recognition led to the placement of the child at the center, with pediatrician, specialists, social workers, and therapists coordinating care around the child's needs. This innovative structure developed into the PCMH model of healthcare delivery now endorsed by the four major professional societies who represent primary care practitioners [155].

H. B. Bosworth, *Enhancing Medication Adherence: The Public Health Dilemma*, DOI: 10.1007/978-1-908517-66-1_5, © Springer Healthcare 2012

These four societies include the American Academy of Family Physicians (AAFP), the American Academy of Pediatrics (AAP), the American College of Physicians (ACP), and the American Osteopathic Association (AOA); national employers and their associations, quality advocacy groups, academic centers, and consumer advocacy groups also currently support the PCMH model.

The essential feature of PCMH is to retain the primacy of an ongoing relationship between patients and their primary care providers. This relationship has been expanded to include other members of a core team, such as clerks and nurses, with whom both the patient and provider have an ongoing relationship. Other providers, including pharmacists, dieticians, and other clinical support staff, can complete the team, depending on the patient's needs. The approach is proactive, both in rigorously assessing for and addressing known risk factors and health issues [156]. One goal for PCMH is to remove barriers, physical and temporal, between the patient and healthcare team. This requires an open-scheduling system, superb communication systems among team members and with the patient, optimal delegation of tasks among team members, enhanced use of nonface-to-face care, and integration of all clinical data by the primary care team. When implemented well, PCMH can improve quality of care and patient and provider satisfaction [156,157]. Further work is needed to assess the role of PCMH in improving medication adherence.

The role of the clinician

Physicians have an important, largely unrealized, opportunity to improve their patients' adherence. Their role begins with awareness of the problem and some type of assessment of adherence in each patient. Providers may need to learn to assess the potential for nonadherence, know the broad determinants of and risk factors for nonadherence, be familiar with proven strategies to improve adherence, and tailor interventions to the needs of individual patients [1]. In addition, providers need to follow evidence-based guidelines and prescribe appropriate medications, since the benefits of adherence are contingent on the benefits of the medications themselves.

Some practical measures that clinicians can implement include screening for missed appointments. Missed appointments correlate with lower adherence rates, and are the first sign of dropping out of care entirely, the most severe form of nonadherence. Telephone or appointment reminders provide relatively easy methods to reduce nonadherence.

Common misperceptions should be anticipated and avoided; for example, that a medication for a chronic condition can be stopped when the prescription runs out or, for largely asymptomatic conditions like hypertension or hyperlipidemia, that medications should only be taken when symptoms arise.

> Common mistakes that clinicians make in communication include overwhelming the patient with too much information, using jargon and technical terminology, relying on words alone, and failing to assess patient understanding [158–160]. Employing effective communication techniques may be one of the most important interventions to reduce health disparities related to low health literacy.

A few studies have specifically examined how physicians communicate the risks and benefits of medications during medical visits [161–163]. Sleath et al investigated physician and patient questions about medications in a sample of 467 audiotaped primary care visits [161]. All patients were on at least one prescribed medication, with an average of four prescribed medications. The researchers found that physicians asked patients about how the medication was working for them during 56% of visits and they asked about side effects during only 27% of visits. Patients asked about side effects during 5% of visits [161].

> " Recommendations for how the healthcare provider can improve health communication include employing patient-centered communication methods, clear communication techniques, confirmation of understanding, and reinforcement [164]. Clinicians should also attempt to prioritize and limit the number of key points discussed to three or fewer [165]. "

At the system level, some helpful interventions for patients with low-health literacy include designing and offering easy-to-understand health educational materials and chronic disease management programs, improving medication drug labeling, creating an empowering environment, and offering communication training to clinicians [164].

Shared-decision making

Shared-decision making (SDM) frames health decisions as an exchange between patient and healthcare provider with two key components [166,167]:
1. The joint identification of advantages and disadvantages of a specific health behavior by the patient and provider.
2. The provision of education about the illness and corresponding treatments.

Various channels have been used to provide this information, with internet applications and social networks being especially promising innovations [168]. SDM is fundamentally a social exchange; thus, counseling skills that enhance engagement are important. Several essential elements [166,167] that physicians can employ for SDM include:

- defining and explaining the problem;
- presenting options;
- discussing pros and cons (eg, benefits, risks, costs);
- eliciting a patient's values and preferences;
- discussing the patient's ability and self-efficacy;
- offering knowledge and recommendations;
- checking and clarifying patient understanding;
- moving or deferring a decision, if needed; and
- arranging follow-up.

Research has examined SDM for a variety of illnesses and disabilities, including treatment decisions related to cancer [169], mental illness [170], and substance abuse [167]. Meta-analyses and reviews of studies yielded mixed conclusions [171,172]. Results showed that SDM leads to enhanced satisfaction with, and more knowledge about, treatments and their providers. Adherence seemed to improve in about one-quarter to as many as two-thirds of research participants, yet improvement in adherence frequently diminished in the weeks after intervention ceased. Moreover, characteristics of research participants, especially as related to their rational capabilities, seemed to diminish effects; however, in studies that have examined actual professional–patient interactions, researchers found that healthcare professionals almost always fail to adequately educate patients and enlist them in a process that meets the criteria for fully informed decision making [173,174].

Motivational interviewing and medication adherence

Motivational interviewing might be viewed as a form of SDM, as it was originally developed as a treatment for substance abuse and later became an adjunct for behaviors associated with other illnesses [175]. Motivational interviewing presumes stages of change that are defined by perceived costs and benefits of a health decision [176]. Using hypertension as an example, patients in what has been called the "contemplation stage" admit to some disadvantages of high blood pressure (eg, risk of worse cardiac illness, reduced mobility, poorer sense of well-being), but believe its actual costs are minimal (eg, patients do not regularly experience bothersome symptoms, they believe that there is no need to disrupt current dietary choices). Alternatively, precontemplation is the stage where patients fail to recognize any costs to a condition (eg, "High blood pressure is not really a problem for me! After all, my father lived with it for years"). Motivational interviewing is a clinical intervention meant to impact stages of change. It expands the simple balance sheet into a counseling process resting on four basic counseling principles [177] similar to SDM:

1. Express empathy.
2. Develop discrepancy.
3. Roll with resistance.
4. Support self-efficacy.

> " Motivational interviewing has been shown to be effective in improving general health status or well-being, promoting physical activity, developing healthier nutritional habits, encouraging medication adherence, and managing chronic conditions, such as mental illness, hypertension, hypercholesterolemia, obesity, and diabetes [178–182]. "

This process is more likely to be successful if the patient has a positive attitude about the need for change. Motivational interviewing is intended to help patients recognize and address their problems and enhance their perception of treatment efficacy [177]. In the case of chronic diseases, such as hypertension, optimal adherence to medications depends largely on the relationship established between the healthcare professional and patient. If the healthcare professional merely issues unilateral declarations about a treatment plan, the patient is less likely to adopt changes that have a positive impact on his or her health. The motivation for change is greater if a patient and his or her healthcare professional work together to make treatment decisions. Additionally, patient outcomes are better if the patient assumes responsibility for his or her own circumstances (local control) [177].

In summary, motivational interviewing has been shown to be equivalent to more intensive treatment, efficacious at low doses (two or three sessions), effective as pretreatment adjunct and as an approach for less motivated or prepared patients, and applicable in a wide range of situations for diverse populations.

The role of the pharmacist

The WHO have advocated for a multidisciplinary approach in addressing nonadherence. In this approach, the community pharmacist can play an important role in ensuring that drug therapy is appropriate [1]. Community pharmacists are among the most easily accessible healthcare providers, have extensive knowledge about drug therapy and disease management, and can provide information and education to the patient and monitor adherence. Direct pharmacy interventions, such as pharmacy continuing medical education developed by pharmaceutical manufacturers and, more recently, packaging manufacturers, have been developed to help optimize pharmacist counseling time and efficiency.

Several RCT have been conducted in which pharmaceutical interventions to enhance medication adherence have been implemented [183–185]. Evaluated interventions range from giving patients more information and education on the goals and benefits of drug therapy to the simplification of the drug regimen and intensification of patient care by telephone reminders, home visits, and follow-up interviews.

As less than optimal medication regimens have been associated with reduced adherence, several approaches have been investigated to improve the processes of care, such as computerized alerts to healthcare providers in the outpatient setting, which appear to have improved processes of care [186,187]. For example, an automatic alert to pharmacists about potentially inappropriate medications, such as amitriptyline and diazepam for elderly patients, led to significant decreases in the dispensing of these medications [186]. In addition, one study noted that an automated alert to healthcare providers increased the ordering of laboratory tests to monitor for potential adverse drug effects [187].

Interactive voice response technology is a computer-based telephone system, which initiates calls, provides information, and collects data from users. Furthermore, studies with interactive voice response telemonitoring interventions have been shown to improve adherence to medications for chronic diseases and intermediate outcomes, such as diastolic blood pressure and hemoglobin A1C levels [188–190].

Chapter 6

Medication intervention recommendations

Addressing medication adherence

Methods that can be used to improve adherence can be grouped into four general categories:

1. Patient education.
2. Improved dosing schedules.
3. Increased hours when the clinic is open (including evening hours) with subsequent shorter wait times.
4. Improved communication between physicians and patients.

> ❝ *Improving medication adherence in the context of chronic diseases can be addressed in three steps. The first step is initiation, followed by adjustment, and then maintenance. Medication adherence management starts with instructing the patient at the initiation of treatment and providing careful monitoring and support during the early treatment stage [191,192].* ❞

For patients who require more than one prescription, medications should be prescribed to be taken at the same time if this is consistent with the appropriate therapeutic activity. When starting a new prescription at the time of hospital discharge – an especially vulnerable transition time in patient care – providing a 1-month supply of all new medications to the patient prior to discharge has been adopted by some successful healthcare programs, including the Geisinger Health System.

H. B. Bosworth, *Enhancing Medication Adherence: The Public Health Dilemma*, DOI: 10.1007/978-1-908517-66-1_6,
© Springer Healthcare 2012

Negotiating a therapy that the patient is able to follow should be a first priority. Besides simplifying the dosing regimen, some examples of ways to tailor the therapy to the individual's needs include exploring the patient's schedule, beliefs and preferences, altering the administration route, and using adherence aids [5,193].

The most common adherence problems encountered at the start of treatment [192] are that the patient:

- lacks knowledge of the disease and its treatment;
- rejects the diagnosis and/or the prescribed drug;
- rejects the prescribed drug;
- lacks the skills to establish self medication as a habit; and
- engages in frequent self-debate decisions regarding whether to follow prescribed regimens.

The five most common strategies for overcoming these adherence problems are [191]:

1. Specifying the problem in concrete terms.
2. Identifying possible solutions.
3. Developing a plan for implementing the solutions.
4. Trying out the solutions.
5. Evaluating the results.

Furthermore, the ability to pay for prescriptions may impact medication adherence; as previously mentioned, in the USA the coverage gap in Part D of Medicare may make some medications too expensive for some patients. Sometimes, generics provided at lower cost can offer a solution.

Less attention has been given to the evaluation of strategies that might be effective at maintaining adherence. The maintenance-directed intervention strategies used most consistently have been educational or behavioral in nature. Educational interventions, involving patients, their family members, or both, can be effective in improving adherence [194]. Decades of research have confirmed that social contexts influence morbidity and mortality [195–197], in part because social support enhances treatment adherence [197–203]. Social support for chronic disease management includes both emotional support (ie, the provision of empathy, feedback, trust, and love) and instrumental support (ie, physical care, transportation, finances, and help with errands). The involvement of others (family, friends, or coworkers) in the knowledge and treatment of the condition is also a critical part of social support, and may be especially important for the self-management of chronic disease, as studies have found marriage is associated with medication adherence [204].

> *Encouraging patients to access social support can play a significant role in the successful initiation of a medication regimen. The goal of social-support strategies is to develop an ally who can help ease the behavioral change, reduce obstacles to maintenance, and be supportive during failures and successes. Social support is also crucial to long-term treatment plans that require continuous action on the part of the patient.*

Combined use of written and verbal instruction may enhance treatment adherence [205]. Written instructions about the medication regimen should be a core part of every interaction with the patient. Written instructions should use short words and general terms (rather than medical jargon), simple sentence structure, active voice, avoidance of abstract concepts, and use of concrete suggestions.

Return demonstration of information (ie, how to take pills) is a way to ensure patients understand relevant information. Package inserts are important for providing risk–benefit information, but often fail to highlight benefits of treatment and have been shown to have little effect on self-reported behavior [206]. It is better to provide limited amounts of materials, and these materials should relate to and reinforce what is covered in the visit [207]. Educational programs should be based on an appraisal of each individual's needs rather than relying upon general information for all. Providers must establish what is known before offering the patient new knowledge. Providers should use concrete examples to support or explain concepts.

Behavioral strategies, including self-monitoring, cueing, chaining (associating new behaviors with established ones), positive reinforcement, and patient contracting have been used to enhance medication adherence [208,209]. In a contingency contract, both providers and patients set forth a treatment goal and their specific obligations in attempting to accomplish this goal, and a time limit for its achievement. A contract may include:

- a written outline of the expected behavior;
- a promise to involve the patient in the decision-making process concerning the treatment regimen;
- the opportunity to discuss potential problems and solutions with the provider;
- a formal commitment to the medical problem from the patient; and
- rewards that create incentives for adherence goals.

Additional strategies include developing prompts and reminder systems, identifying potential relapses into old behavior, setting appropriate and realistic goals, and rewarding achievement of new behaviors. Maintenance of most behaviors declines over time; therefore, constant questioning and follow-up are essential to ensure adequate adherence [117].

Some specific behavior recommendations for medication adherence include:

1. Using medication-reminder cues and placing medication taking within patients' habitual daily routines. The cues can be activities, such as personal toilet routines, meals, coffee, or bedtime. An example of a physical cue is the medication container placed prominently by a patient's toothbrush; every time an individual may brush their teeth at night, they will be then reminded to take their medication.

2. Patients should receive a written medication description with instructions on starting the prescription. This includes the drug's name, strength, and form; the medical conditions treated or purpose of medication; the number of doses per day and their time of day; the relationship to food, beverages, and other medications; and any special instructions for responding to potential drug–drug interactions.

3. Patients should be encouraged to maintain a daily medication record of each dose taken or missed with relevant comments.

The clinician or appropriate member of the healthcare team can review this medication diary with the patient over the telephone or at the next clinic visit.

Goal setting must be implemented as part of the initiation of the treatment regimen. Working toward a goal that is specific, attainable, and proximal in time heightens self-efficacy and promotes behavioral change. A time frame should be included in the goals (eg, in 2 weeks or at the time of the next visit in 4 weeks). Telephone contacts may be used to review progress toward the goal when the patient is not seen on a frequent basis. When the goal is attained, reinforcement is provided for the success, and the next level of the goals is set. When the patient is unsuccessful in attaining the behavior, the provider can encourage the patient to continue. Additionally, by utilizing the latest medical technology, patients could be empowered in a novel way to promote self-management of their chronic conditions, beginning with better management of their medication adherence.

Dosing schedules

Strategies to improve dosing schedules include the use of pillboxes to organize daily doses, simplifying the regimen to daily dosing, and cues to remind patients to take medications. There is an increasing number of products being introduced into the market to assist individuals with organizing their medications. A fundamental component of all these devices is the knowledge of how to initially organize their medications. Thus, for children or those with cognitive impairments, pillboxes may not be appropriate. In addition, newer medications are entering the market that are either combination medications or require less frequent dosing because of longer half-lives; however, these medications are typically more costly and less likely to be covered by insurance. In terms of the combination medications there is also a need to be cautious regarding over-medicating.

Patient–provider communication

Enhancing communication between the physician and patient is a key and effective strategy in boosting the patient's ability to follow a medication regimen [210,211]; however, education and training of medical personnel in adherence diagnosis and management is not always readily available in current medical education. Authoritative textbooks on general medicine, medical therapies, pharmacology, and patient interviewing do not typically address adherence and its management. Drug-industry publications for healthcare professionals occasionally have brief descriptions of the rudiments of adherence management. However, most clinicians learn adherence management simply through clinical experience. A variety of healthcare personnel can be trained to assist clinicians as effective adherence counselors, including nurses, physician's assistants, dietitians, psychologists, and office staff.

> *Behaviors, such as a provider making direct eye contact, transmitting interest in what the patient says, explaining recommendations thoroughly and clearly, praising treatment adherence and problem solving, and expressing willingness to modify the treatment plan in accordance with the patient's concerns, have been demonstrated as ways to promote adherence [212]. Additional methods to improve the interaction of the provider with patients include expressing empathy and acceptance through the use of active listening and reflective responses. Providers should also resist entering into conflict with the patient and avoid the imposition of their own values or beliefs onto the patient.*

Patients should be provided with a clear rationale for the necessity of a particular treatment and their concerns should be elicited and addressed. To ensure that the necessary information has been understood, key instructions should be provided both verbally and in written form and the patient should be asked to verify that they understand the instructions [213]. Common misperceptions should be anticipated and avoided, including that the medication can be stopped when the prescription runs out or when the condition comes under control, different medications cannot be taken together at the same time of the day, or that symptoms are guides to when to take medication. In addition, use of medical jargon may leave patients feeling disengaged and devoid of responsibility for their care; thus, it is important for physicians to speak to their patients in layperson terms when discussing their medications and medication plan.

Organizational issues

Missing appointments is correlated with lower adherence rates to prescribed regimens, and is the first sign of dropping out of care entirely, the most severe form of nonadherence. Patients who miss appointments are often those who need the most help in improving their ability to adhere to a medication regimen. Relatively easy methods to overcome this problem include using appointment reminders by letter or telephone, contracting with patients to keep appointments, and contacting patients immediately if appointments are missed. Calling patients who miss appointments is logically the most important method for helping patients adhere to prescribed regimens because reminding or recalling patients is effective and relatively inexpensive [214]. Additional organizational factors include making follow-up visits convenient and efficient for the patient; for example, delays in seeing patients and problems with transportation and parking can undermine a patient's willingness to adhere with a medication regimen and to keep follow-up appointments.

For healthcare systems in which pharmacy records are readily available, a review of the refill frequency and the date of the last refill may also help identify nonadherence. Once medication nonadherence is recognized, healthcare providers and patients can work collaboratively to develop patient-specific solutions to address adherence barriers. Interventions that enlist ancillary healthcare providers, such as pharmacists, behavioral specialists, and nursing staff, can also help improve adherence.

Finally, enhancing communication between the physician and the patient is a key and effective strategy in boosting the patient's ability to follow a medication regimen. Most methods of improving adherence have involved combinations of behavioral interventions and reinforcements in addition to increasing the convenience of care, providing educational information about the patient's condition and the treatment, and other forms of supervision or attention. Successful methods tend to be complex and labor intensive; innovative strategies will need to be developed that are practical for routine clinical use.

66 *Given the many factors contributing to poor adherence to medication, a multifactorial approach is required, since a single approach will not be effective for all patients.* **99**

Chapter 7

Future directions and recommendations

There are both enormous challenges and opportunities in addressing the public health crisis of medication adherence. One important theme is that the multifactorial basis for nonadherence calls for a multifaceted solution. An initial step is a common understanding of some of the key issues among stakeholders and the need to routinely measure and track adherence in standard practice. Electronic health systems provide an important opportunity to address that gap, particularly with guidance from the HHS on defining meaningful use to include measurement and integration of tools that improve adherence within EHRs.

Providers need to receive further training on screening and resolving nonadherence as well. In general, patients tend to overestimate their medication adherence [117], and unless a patient is not responding to therapy, it may be extremely difficult to identify poor medication adherence. Asking patients about their medication use is often the most practical means of ascertainment, but it is prone to inaccuracy. Other practical measures to assess adherence include seeing if patients do not respond to increments in treatment intensity and noting those who fail to attend appointments. Additional practical methods include review of pill bottles, and, when available, checking fill dates and pill counts. Finally, simply asking the patient to describe their medication regimen, such as when they take their medication and what the medications are for, can often be very informative. Poor adherence should always be considered when a patient's condition is not responding to therapy. Patients should also be

H. B. Bosworth, *Enhancing Medication Adherence: The Public Health Dilemma*, DOI: 10.1007/978-1-908517-66-1_7, © Springer Healthcare 2012

asked whether they are having any side effects from their medications, whether they know why they are taking their medications, and what the benefits of taking them are, since an inability to answer these questions adequately can often expose poor adherence to a regimen [109].

> **❝** An ideal system for improving adherence would not only engage the patient themselves, but also leverage their selected healthcare providers, caregivers, and communal support network. **❞**

Conclusion

In summary, if over 100 different factors have been identified as potential predictors of medication adherence, one cannot expect a "one size fits all" intervention strategy. For instance, technology will increase in use and will likely help many individuals, but development of technology needs continued input from both patients and providers on how to incorporate these advances into clinical care. We need to examine alternative methods of implementing interventions; ideally, through a readily available and easy-to-use "toolbox" for which providers receive adequate training in its use. Reimbursement models for medication adherence is an additional avenue that is worth further exploration.

References

1   Sabate E. World Health Organization. Adherence to long-term therapies: evidence for action. www.who.int/chp/knowledge/publications/adherence_introduction.pdf. Published 2003. Accesssed February 28, 2012.

2   Osterberg L, Blaschke T. Adherence to medication. *N Engl J Med*. 2005;353:487-497.

3   Benner JS, Glynn RJ, Mogun H, Neumann PJ, Weinstein MC, Avorn J. Long-term persistence in use of statin therapy in elderly patients. *JAMA*. 2002;288:455-461.

4   Avorn J, Monette J, Lacour A, et al. Persistence of use of lipid-lowering medications: a cross-national study. *JAMA*. 1998;279:1458-1462.

5   Feldman R, Bacher M, Campbell N, Drover A, Chockalingam A. Adherence to pharmacologic management of hypertension. *Can J Public Health*. 1998;89:I16-I18.

6   Flack J, Novikov SV, Ferrario CM. Benefits of adherence to antihypertensive drug therapy. *Eur Heart J*. 1996;17(Suppl A):16-20.

7   Mallion JM, Baguet JP, Siche JP, Tremel F, de Gaudemaris R. Compliance, electronic monitoring and antihypertensive drugs. *J Hypertens Suppl*. 1998;16:S75-S79.

8   Haynes RB, McKibbon KA, Kanani R. Systematic review of randomised trials of interventions to assist patients to follow prescriptions for medications. *Lancet*. 1996;348:383-386.

9   National Council on Patient Information and Education. Enhancing prescription medication adherence: a national action plan. www.talkaboutrx.org/documents/enhancing_prescription_medicine_adherence.pdf. Published August 2007. Accessed February 28, 2012.

10 Sherman FT. Medication nonadherence: a national epidemic among America's seniors. *Geriatrics*. 2007;62:5-6.

11 McCarthy R. The price you pay for the drug not taken. *Bus Health*. 1998;16:27-33.

12 Haynes RB, Ackloo E, Sahota N, McDonald HP, Yao X. Interventions for enhancing medication adherence. *Cochrane Database Syst Rev*. 2008;(2):CD000011.

13 Stuart BC, Simoni-Wastila L, Zhao L, Lloyd JT, Doshi JA. Increased persistency in medication use by U.S. Medicare beneficiaries with diabetes is associated with lower hospitalization rates and cost savings. *Diabetes Care*. 2009;32:647-649.

14 Stuart B, Davidoff A, Lopert R, Shaffer T, Samantha Shoemaker J, Lloyd J. Does medication adherence lower Medicare spending among beneficiaries with diabetes? *Health Serv Res*. 2011;46:1180-1199.

15 Stuart B, Simoni-Wastila L, Yin X, Davidoff A, Zuckerman IH, Doshi J. Medication use and adherence among elderly Medicare beneficiaries with diabetes enrolled in Part D and retiree health plans. *Med Care*. 2011;49:511-515.

16 Mahoney JJ. Reducing patient drug acquisition costs can lower diabetes health claims. *Am J Manag Care*. 2005;11:S170-S176.

17 Cramer JA, Roy A, Burrell A, et al. Medication compliance and persistence: terminology and definitions. *Value Health*. 2008;11:44-47.

18 Bosworth H, Granger BB, Mendys P, et al. Medication adherence: a call for action. *Am Heart J*. 2001;162:412-424.

19 Haynes RB, Yao X, Degani A, Kripalani S, Garg A, McDonald HP. Interventions to enhance medication adherence. *Cochrane Database Syst Rev*. 2005;(4):CD000011.

20 Jackevicius CA, Li P, Tu JV. Prevalence, predictors, and outcomes of primary nonadherence after acute myocardial infarction. *Circulation*. 2008;117:1028-1036.

H. B. Bosworth, *Enhancing Medication Adherence: The Public Health Dilemma*, DOI: 10.1007/978-1-908517-66-1, © Springer Healthcare 2012

21   Raebel MA, Ellis JL, Carroll NM, et al. Characteristics of patients with primary non-adherence to medications for hypertension, diabetes, and lipid disorders. *J Gen Intern Med*. 2011;27:57-64.

22   Raebel MA, Carroll NM, Ellis JL, Schroeder EB, Bayliss EA. Importance of including early nonadherence in estimations of medication adherence. *Ann Pharmacother*. 2011;45:1053-1060.

23   Rasmussen JN, Chong A, Alter DA. Relationship between adherence to evidence-based pharmacotherapy and long-term mortality after acute myocardial infarction. *JAMA*. 2007;297:177-186.

24   Lehane E, McCarthy G. An examination of the intentional and unintentional aspects of medication non-adherence in patients diagnosed with hypertension. *J Clin Nurs*. 2007;16:698-706.

25   Rudd P. Clinicians and patients with hypertension: unsettled issues about compliance. *Am Heart J*. 1995;130:572-579.

26   Kruse W, Koch-Gwinner P, Nikolaus T, Oster P, Schlierf G, Weber E. Measurement of drug compliance by continuous electronic monitoring: a pilot study in elderly patients discharged from hospital. *J Am Geriatr Soc*. 1992;40:1151-1155.

27   Thorpe CT, Bryson CL, Maciejewski ML, Bosworth HB. Medication acquisition and self-reported adherence in veterans with hypertension. *Med Care*. 2009;47:474-481.

28   Nikolaus T, Kruse W, Bach M, Specht-Leible N, Oster P, Schlierf G. Elderly patients' problems with medication. An in-hospital and follow-up study. *Eur J Clin Pharmacol*. 1996;49:255-259.

29   Lowe CJ, Raynor DK, Courtney EA, Purvis J, Teale C. Effects of self medication programme on knowledge of drugs and compliance with treatment in elderly patients. *BMJ*. 1995;310:1229-1231.

30   Bender BG, Bender SE. Patient-identified barriers to asthma treatment adherence responses to interviews, focus groups, and questionnaires. *Immunol Allergy Clin N Am*. 2005;25:107-130.

31   Esposito L. The effects of medication education on adherence to medication regimens in an elderly population. *J Adv Nurs*. 1995;21:935-943.

32   Lawrence J, Mayers DL, Hullsiek KH, et al. Structured treatment interruption in patients with multidrug-resistant human immunodeficiency virus. *N Engl J Med*. 2003;349:837-846.

33   Park D. Applied cognitive aging research. In: Craik FIM, Salthouse TA, ed. *The Handbook of Aging and Cognition*. Hillsdale, NJ: Lawrence Erlbaum; 1992:449-493.

34   Park D, Kidder DP. Prospective memory and medication adherence. In: Brandimonte MGE, McDaniel MA, ed. *Prospective Memory Theory and Application*. Hillsdale, NJ: Lawrence Erlbaum; 1996:369-390.

35   Bosworth HB, Schaie KW. Medication knowledge and health status in the Seattle Longitudinal Study. In: Ryan EG, Berg C, chairs. *Cognition: Clinical Issues*. Annual Meeting of Geronotological Society of America, Los Angeles, CA. www.uwpsychiatry.org/sls/Med%20know%20hlth%20 stat%20in%20SLS.pdf. Published November 1995. Accessed February 28, 2012.

36   Salthouse T. *Theoretical Perspectives in Cognitive Aging*. Hillsdale, NJ: Lawrence Erlbaum; 1991.

37   Farmer ME, Kittner SJ, Abbott RD, Wolz MM, Wolf PA, White LR. Longitudinally measured blood pressure, antihypertensive medication use, and cognitive performance: the Framingham Study. *J Clin Epidemiol*. 1990;43:475-480.

38   Wilson IB, Tchetgen E, Spiegelman D. Patterns of adherence with antiretroviral medications: an examination of between-medication differences. *J Acquir Immune Defic Syndr*. 2001;28:259-263.

39   Salzman C. Medication compliance in the elderly. *J Clin Psychiatry*. 1995;56:18-22.

40   Berg JS, Dischler J, Wagner DJ, Raia JJ, Palmer-Shevlin N. Medication compliance: a healthcare problem. *Ann Pharmacother*. 1993;27:S1-S24.

41   Cameron C. Patient compliance: recognition of factors involved and suggestions for promoting compliance with therapeutic regimens. *J Adv Nurs*. 1996;24:244-250.

42   Bosworth HB. *Improving Patient Treatment Adherence: A Clinician Guidebook*. New York, NY: Springer; 2010.

43   Peterson AM, Takiya L, Finley R. Meta-analysis of trials of interventions to improve medication adherence. *Am J Health Syst Pharm*. 2003;60:657-665.

44   Glynn LG, Murphy AW, Smith SM, Schroeder K, Fahey T. Interventions used to improve control of blood pressure in patients with hypertension. *Cochrane Database Syst Rev*. 2010;(3):CD005182.

45   Vermeire E, Hearnshaw H, Van Royen P, Denekens J. Patient adherence to treatment: three decades of research. A comprehensive review. *J Clin Pharm Ther*. 2001;26:331-342.

46   Marx G, Witte N, Himmel W, Kuhnel S, Simmenroth-Nayda A, Koschack J. Accepting the unacceptable: Medication adherence and different types of action patterns among patients with high blood pressure. *Patient Educ Couns*. 2011;85:468-474.

47   Haynes R, Taylor DW, Sackett DL. *Compliance in Healthcare*. Baltimore, MD: John Hopkins University Press; 1978.

48   Cramer J, Spilker B. *Patient Compliance in Medical Practice and Clinical Trials*. New York: Raven Press; 1991.

49   Haynes RB, Taylor DW, Sackett DL. *Compliance in Healthcare*. Baltimore, MD: Johns Hopkins University Press; 1981.

50   Gorman AA, Foley FM, Ettenhofer MI, Hinkin CH, van Gorp WG. Functional consequences of HIV-associated neuropsychological impairment. *Neuropsychol Rev*. 2009;19:186-203.

51   Williams A, Manias E, Walker R. Interventions to improve medication adherence in people with multiple chronic conditions: a systematic review. *J Adv Nurs*. 2008;63:132-143.

52   Powers B, Bosworth HB. Revisiting literacy and adherence: Future clinical and research directions. *J Gen Intern Med*. 2006;21:1341-1342.

53   Pignone MP, DeWalt DA. Literacy and health outcomes: is adherence the missing link? *J Gen Intern Med*. 2006;21:896-897.

54   Schroeder K, Fahey T, Ebrahim S. Interventions for improving adherence to treatment in patients with high blood pressure in ambulatory settings. *Cochrane Database Syst Rev*. 2004;(2):CD004804.

55   Schedlbauer A, Schroeder K, Fahey T. How can adherence to lipid-lowering medication be improved? A systematic review of randomized controlled trials. *Fam Pract*. 2007;24:380-387.

56   Gold DT, Alexander IM, Ettinger MP. How can osteoporosis patients benefit more from their therapy? Adherence issues with bisphosphonate therapy. *Ann Pharmacother*. 2006;40:1143-1150.

57   Chia LR, Schlenk EA, Dunbar-Jacob J. Effect of personal and cultural beliefs on medication adherence in the elderly. *Drugs Aging*. 2006;23:191-202.

58   Gallant MP. The influence of social support on chronic illness self-management: a review and directions for research. *Health Educ Behav*. 2003;30:170-195.

59   DiMatteo MR, Lepper HS, Croghan TW. Depression is a risk factor for noncompliance with medical treatment: meta-analysis of the effects of anxiety and depression on patient adherence. *Arch Intern Med*. 2000;160:2101-2107.

60   Nair KV, Belletti DA, Doyle JJ, et al. Understanding barriers to medication adherence in the hypertensive population by evaluating responses to a telephone survey. *Patient Prefer Adherence*. 2011;5:195-206.

61   McCray AT. Promoting health literacy. *J Am Med Inform Assoc*. 2005;12:152-163.

62   Institute of Medicine. *Health literacy. A prescription to End Confusion*. Washington, DC: National Academies Press; 2004.

63   US Department of Education. National Assessment of Adult Literacy. A first look at the literacy of America's adults in the 21st century. nces.ed.gov/naal/pdf/2006470.pdf. Published 2005. Accessed February 28, 2012.

64   Gazmararian JA, Baker DW, Williams MV, et al. Health literacy among Medicare enrollees in a managed care organization. *JAMA*. 1999;281:545-551.

65   Williams M, Parker RM, Baker DW, et al. Inadequate functional health literacy among patients at two public hospitals. *JAMA*. 1995;274:1677-1682.

66   Wilson FL, Racine E, Tekieli V, Williams B. Literacy, readability and cultural barriers: critical factors to consider when educating older African Americans about anticoagulation therapy. *J Clin Nurs*. 2003;12:275-282.

67   Nelson W, Reyna VF, Fagerlin A, Lipkus I, Peters E. Clinical implications of numeracy: theory and practice. *Ann Behav Med*. 2008;35:261-274.

68   Gazmararian JA, Williams MV, Peel J, Baker DW. Health literacy and knowledge of chronic disease. *Patient Educ Couns*. 2003;51:267-275.

69   Parker RM, Gazmararian JA. Health literacy: essential for health communication. *J Health Commun*. 2003;8(Suppl 1):116-118.

70   Powers BJ, Trinh JV, Bosworth HB. Can this patient read and understand written health information? *JAMA*. 2010;304:76-84.

71   Hauptman PJ. Medication adherence in heart failure. *Heart Fail Rev*. 2008;13:99-106.

72   Bodenheimer T, Lorig K, Holman H, Grumbach K. Patient self-management of chronic disease in primary care. *JAMA*. 2002;288:2469-2475.

73   Jerant AF, von Friederichs-Fitzwater MM, Moore M. Patients' perceived barriers to active self-management of chronic conditions. *Patient Educ Couns*. 2005;57:300-307.

74   Bayliss EA, Steiner JF, Fernald DH, Crane LA, Main DS. Descriptions of barriers to self-care by persons with comorbid chronic diseases. *Ann Fam Med*. 2003;1:15-21.

75   Williams A. Patients with comorbidities: perceptions of acute care services. *J Adv Nurs*. 2004;46:13-22.

76   Williams B, Shaw A, Durrant R, Crinson I, Pagliari C, de Lusignan S. Patient perspectives on multiple medications versus combined pills: a qualitative study. *QJM*. 2005;98:885-893.

77   Pound P, Britten N, Morgan M, et al. Resisting medicines: a synthesis of qualitative studies of medicine taking. *Soc Sci Med*. 2005;61:133-155.

78   Tarn DM, Heritage J, Paterniti DA, Hays RD, Kravitz RL, Wenger NS. Physician communication when prescribing new medications. *Arch Intern Med*. 2006;166:1855-1862.

79   Thinking outside the pillbox: A system-wide approach to improving patient medication adherence for chronic disease. New England Healthcare Institute. www.nehi.net/publications/44/thinking_outside_the_pillbox_a_systemwide. Published August 12, 2009. Accessed February 28, 2012.

80   Goldman DP, Joyce GF, Zheng Y. Prescription drug cost sharing: associations with medication and medical utilization and spending and health. *JAMA*. 2007;298:61-69.

81   Piette JD, Heisler M, Wagner TH. Cost-related medication underuse: do patients with chronic illnesses tell their doctors? *Arch Intern Med*. 2004;164:1749-1755.

82   Piette JD, Heisler M, Krein S, Kerr EA. The role of patient-physician trust in moderating medication nonadherence due to cost pressures. *Arch Intern Med*. 2005;165:1749-1755.

83   Doshi JA, Zhu J, Lee BY, Kimmel SE, Volpp KG. Impact of a prescription copayment increase on lipid-lowering medication adherence in veterans. *Circulation*. 2009;119:390-397.

84   Soumerai SB, Pierre-Jacques M, Zhang F, et al. Cost-related medication nonadherence among elderly and disabled medicare beneficiaries: a national survey 1 year before the medicare drug benefit. *Arch Intern Med*. 2006;166:1829-1835.

85   Hsu J, Price M, Huang J, et al. Unintended consequences of caps on Medicare drug benefits. *N Engl J Med*. 2006;354:2349-2359.

86   Thorpe KE. Cost sharing, caps on benefits, and the chronically ill—a policy mismatch. *N Engl J Med*. 2006;354:2385-2386.

87   Maciejewski ML, Bryson CL, Perkins M, et al. Increasing copayments and adherence to diabetes, hypertension, and hyperlipidemic medications. *Am J Manag Care*. 2010;16:e20-e34.

88   Heisler M, Choi H, Rosen AB, et al. Hospitalizations and deaths among adults with cardiovascular disease who underuse medications because of cost: a longitudinal analysis. *Med Care*. 2010;48:87-94.

89   Zeber JE, Grazier KL, Valenstein M, Blow FC, Lantz PM. Effect of a medication copayment increase in veterans with schizophrenia. *Am J Manag Care*. 2007;13:335-346.

90 Fendrick AM, Chernew ME, Levi GW. Value-based insurance design: embracing value over cost alone. *Am J Manag Care*. 2009;15:S277-S283.

91 Chernew ME, Shah MR, Wegh A, et al. Impact of decreasing copayments on medication adherence within a disease management environment. *Health Aff (Millwood)*. 2008;27:103-112.

92 Choudhry NK, Fischer MA, Avorn J, et al. At Pitney Bowes, value-based insurance design cut copayments and increased drug adherence. *Health Aff (Millwood)*. 2010;29:1995-2001.

93 Shrank WH, Hoang T, Ettner SL, et al. The implications of choice: prescribing generic or preferred pharmaceuticals improves medication adherence for chronic conditions. *Arch Intern Med*. 2006;166:332-337.

94 Volpp KG, Troxel AB, Pauly MV, et al. A randomized, controlled trial of financial incentives for smoking cessation. *N Engl J Med*. 2009;360:699-709.

95 Volpp KG, John LK, Troxel AB, Norton L, Fassbender J, Loewenstein G. Financial incentive-based approaches for weight loss: a randomized trial. *JAMA*. 2008;300:2631-2637.

96 Committee on Quality of Healthcare in America. *Crossing the Quality Chasm: A New Health System for the 21st Century*. Washington, DC: National Academies Press; 2001.

97 Ho PM, Bryson CL, Rumsfeld JS. Medication adherence: its importance in cardiovascular outcomes. *Circulation*. 2009;119:3028-3035.

98 Fonarow GC, Peterson ED. Heart failure performance measures and outcomes: real or illusory gains. *JAMA*. 2009;302:792-794.

99 Patterson ME, Hernandez AF, Hammill BG, et al. Process of care performance measures and long-term outcomes in patients hospitalized with heart failure. *Med Care*. 2010;48:210-216.

100 Peterson ED, Roe MT, Rumsfeld JS, et al. A call to ACTION (acute coronary treatment and intervention outcomes network): a national effort to promote timely clinical feedback and support continuous quality improvement for acute myocardial infarction. *Circ Cardiovasc Qual Outcomes*. 2009;2:491-499.

101 Pillittere-Dugan D, Nau DP, McDonough K, Pierre Z. Development and testing of performance measures for pharmacy services. *J Am Pharm Assoc (2003)*. 2009;49:212-219.

102 Alcoba M, Cuevas MJ, Perez-Simon MR, et al. Assessment of adherence to triple antiretroviral treatment including indinavir: role of the determination of plasma levels of indinavir. *J Acquir Immune Defic Syndr*. 2003;33:253-258.

103 Wagner JH, Justice AC, Chesney M, Sinclair G, Weissman S, Rodriguez-Barradas M. Patient- and provider-reported adherence: toward a clinically useful approach to measuring antiretroviral adherence. *J Clin Epidemiol*. 2001;54:S91-S98.

104 Corrigan P. How stigma interferes with mental health care. *Am Psych*. 2004;59:614-625.

105 Stephenson BJ, Rowe BH, Haynes RB, Macharia WM, Leon G. Is this patient taking the treatment as prescribed? *JAMA*. 1993;269:2779-2781.

106 Choo PW, Rand CS, Inui TS, et al. Validation of patient reports, automated pharmacy records, and pill counts with electronic monitoring of adherence to antihypertensive therapy. *Med Care*. 1999;37:846-857.

107 Steiner JF, Prochazka AV. The assessment of refill compliance using pharmacy records: methods, validity, and applications. *J Clin Epidemiol*. 1997;50:105-116.

108 Rosen MI, Rigsby MO, Salahi JT, Ryan CE, Cramer JA. Electronic monitoring and counseling to improve medication adherence. *Behav Res Ther*. 2004;42:409-422.

109 Morisky E, Green LW, Levine DM. Concurrent and predictive validity of a self-reported measure of medication adherence. *Med Care*. 1986;24:67-74.

110 Thorpe C, Bryson CL, Maciejewski ML, Bosworth HB. Medication acquisition and self-reported adherence in veterans with hypertension. *Med Care*. 2009;47:474-481

111 Shi L, Liu J, Fonseca V, Walker P, Kalsekar A, Pawaskar M. Correlation between adherence rates measured by MEMS and self-reported questionnaires: a meta-analysis. *Health Quality Life Outcomes*. 2010;8:99-104.

112 Morgan AL, Masoudi FA, Havranek EP, et al. Difficulty taking medications, depression, and health status in heart failure patients. *J Cardiac Fail*. 2006;12:54-60.

113 Hansen RA, Kim MM, Song L, Tu W, Wu J, Murray MD. Comparison of methods to assess medication adherence and classify nonadherence. *Ann Pharmacother*. 2009;43:413-422.

114 Krousel-Wood M, Thomas S, Muntner P, Morisky D. Medication adherence: a key factor in achieving blood pressure control and good clinical outcomes in hypertensive patients. *Curr Opin Cardiol*. 2004;19:357-362.

115 Ogedegbe G, Mancuso CA, Allegrante JP, Charlson ME. Development and evaluation of a medication adherence self-efficacy scale in hypertensive African-American patients. *J Clin Epidemiol*. 2003;56:520-529.

116 Ogedegbe G, Harrison M, Robbins L, Mancuso CA, Allegrante JP. Barriers and facilitators of medication adherence in hypertensive African Americans: a qualitative study. *Ethn Dis*. 2004;14:3-12.

117 Dunbar-Jacob J, Dwyer, K, Dunning EJ. Compliance with antihypertensive regimen: A review of the research in the 1980s. *Ann Behav Med*. 1991;13:31-39.

118 Haynes RB, McDonald HP, Garg AX. Helping patients follow prescribed treatment: clinical applications. *JAMA*. 2002;288:2880-2883.

119 Stephenson BJ, Rowe BH, Haynes RB, Macharia WM, Leon G. The rational clinical examination. Is this patient taking the treatment as prescribed? *JAMA*. 1993;269:2779-2781.

120 Simoni JM, Kurth AE, Pearson CR, Pantalone DW, Merrill JO, Frick PA. Self-report measures of antiretroviral therapy adherence: A review with recommendations for HIV research and clinical management. *AIDS Behav*. 2006;10:227-245.

121 Ingersoll KS, Cohen J. The impact of medication regimen factors on adherence to chronic treatment: a review of literature. *J Behav Med*. 2008;31:213-224.

122 Garber MC, Nau DP, Erickson SR, Aikens JE, Lawrence JB. The concordance of self-report with other measures of medication adherence: a summary of the literature. *Med Care*. 2004;42:649-652.

123 Voils CI, Hoyle RH, Thorpe CT, Maciejewski ML, Yancy WS, Jr. Improving the measurement of self-reported medication nonadherence. *J Clin Epidemiol*. 2011;64:250-254.

124 Shalansky SJ, Levy AR, Ignaszewski AP. Self-reported Morisky score for identifying nonadherence with cardiovascular medications. *Ann Pharmacother*. 2004;38:1363-1368.

125 Morisky DE, Ang A, Krousel-Wood M, Ward HJ. Predictive validity of a medication adherence measure in an outpatient setting. *J Clin Hypertens (Greenwich)*. 2008;10:348-354.

126 McHorney CA. The Adherence Estimator: a brief, proximal screener for patient propensity to adhere to prescription medications for chronic disease. *Curr Med Res Opin*. 2009;25:215-238.

127 Stroupe KT, Murray MD, Stump TE, Callahan CM. Association between medication supplies and healthcare costs in older adults from an urban healthcare system. *J Am Geriatr Soc*. 2000;48:760-768.

128 Stroupe KT, Teal EY, Tu W, Weiner M, Murray MD. Association of refill adherence and health care use among adults with hypertension in an urban health care system. *Pharmacother*. 2006;26:779-789.

129 Stroupe KT, Teal EY, Weiner M, Gradus-Pizlo I, Brater DC, Murray MD. Health care and medication costs and use among older adults with heart failure. *Am J Med*. 2004;116:443-450.

130 Yang M, Barner JC, Worchel J. Factors related to antipsychotic oversupply among Central Texas Veterans. *Clin Ther*. 2007;29:1214-1225.

131 Rudd P, Ahmed S, Zachary V, Barton C, Bonduelle D. Improved compliance measures: applications in an ambulatory hypertensive drug trial. *Clin Pharmacol Ther*. 1990;48:676-685.

132 Kimmerling M, Wagner G, Ghosh-Dastidar B. Factors associated with accurate self-reported adherence to HIV antiretrovirals. *Int J STD AIDS*. 2003;14:281-284.

133 Waltherhouse DM, Calzone KA, Mele C, Brenner DE. Adherence to oral tamoxifen: A comparison of patient self report, pill counts and microelectronic monitoring. *J Clin Oncol*. 1993;11:2547-2548.

134 Pullar T, Birtwell AJ, Wiles PG, Hay A, Feely MP. Use of a pharmacologic indicator to compare compliance with tablets prescribed to be taken once, twice, or three times daily. *Clin Pharmacol Ther*. 1988;44:540-545.

135 Maenpaa H, Javela K, Pikkarainen J, Malkonen M, Heinonen OP, Manninen V. Minimal doses of digoxin: a new marker for compliance to medication. *Eur Heart J*. 1987;8(Suppl I):31-37.

136 Gourevitch MN, Wasserman W, Panero MS, Selwyn PA. Successful adherence to observed prophylaxis and treatment of tuberculosis among drug users in a methadone program. *J Addict Dis*. 1996;15:93-104.

137 Volmink J, Garner P. Interventions for promoting adherence to tuberculosis management. *Cochrane Database Syst Rev*. 2000;(4):CD000010.

138 Vermeire E, Wens J, Van Royen P, Biot Y, Hearnshaw H, Lindenmeyer A. Interventions for improving adherence to treatment recommendations in people with type 2 diabetes mellitus. *Cochrane Database Syst Rev*. 2005;(2):CD003638.

139 Rueda S, Park-Wyllie LY, Bayoumi AM, et al. Patient support and education for promoting adherence to highly active antiretroviral therapy for HIV/AIDS. *Cochrane Database Syst Rev*. 2006;(3):CD001442.

140 Heneghan CJ, Glasziou P, Perera R. Reminder packaging for improving adherence to self-administered long-term medications. *Cochrane Database Syst Rev*. 2006;(1):CD005025.

141 Aspden P, Wolcott J, Bootman J, Cronenwett LR, ed. *Preventing Medication Errors*. Washington, DC: Institute of Medicine; 2007.

142 Newby LK, LaPointe NM, Chen AY, et al. Long-term adherence to evidence-based secondary prevention therapies in coronary artery disease. *Circulation*. 2006;113:203-212.

143 Jackevicius CA, Mamdani M, Tu JV. Adherence with statin therapy in elderly patients with and without acute coronary syndromes. *JAMA*. 2002;288:462-467.

144 Makaryus AN, Friedman EA. Patients' understanding of their treatment plans and diagnosis at discharge. *Mayo Clin Proc*. 2005;80:991-994.

145 Coleman EA, Mahoney E, Parry C. Assessing the quality of preparation for posthospital care from the patient's perspective: the care transitions measure. *Med Care*. 2005;43:246-255.

146 Schnipper JL, Kirwin JL, Cotugno MC, et al. Role of pharmacist counseling in preventing adverse drug events after hospitalization. *Arch Intern Med*. 2006;166:565-571.

147 Baroletti S, Dell'Orfano H. Medication adherence in cardiovascular disease. *Circulation*. 2010;121:1455-1458.

148 Cleland JG, Ekman I. Enlisting the help of the largest health care workforce—patients. *JAMA*. 2010;304:1383-1384.

149 The Office of the National Coordinator for Health Information Technology. Electronic Health Records and Meaningful Use. healthit.hhs.gov/portal/server.pt/community/healthit_hhs_gov__meaningful_use_announcement/2996. Last updated February 9, 2011. Accessed February 28, 2012.

150 Centers for Medicare & Medicaid Services. Medicare & Medicaid HER Incentive Program Meaningful Use Stage 1 Requirements Overview. www.cms.gov/EHRIncentivePrograms/Downloads/MU_Stage1_ReqOverview.pdf. Published 2010. Accesssed February 28, 2012.

151 Zedler BK, Kakad P, Colilla S, Murrelle L, Shah NR. Does packaging with a calendar feature improve adherence to self-administered medication for long-term use? A systematic review. *Clin Ther*. 2011;33:62-73.

152 Cutrona SL, Choudhry NK, Stedman M, et al. Physician effectiveness in interventions to improve cardiovascular medication adherence: a systematic review. *J Gen Intern Med*. 2010;25:1090-1096.

153 Carter BL, Rogers M, Daly J, Zheng S, James PA. The potency of team-based care interventions for hypertension: a meta-analysis. *Arch Intern Med*. 2009;169:1748-1755.

154 Carter BL, Bergus GR, Dawson JD, et al. A cluster randomized trial to evaluate physician/pharmacist collaboration to improve blood pressure control. *J Clin Hypertens (Greenwich)*. 2008;10:260-271.

155 Currell R, Urquhart C, Wainwright P, Lewis R. Telemedicine versus face to face patient care: effects on professional practice and health care outcomes. *Cochrane Database Syst Rev.* 2000;(2):CD002098.

156 Reid RJ, Fishman PA, Yu O, et al. Patient-centered medical home demonstration: a prospective, quasi-experimental, before and after evaluation. *Am J Manag Care.* 2009;15:e71-e87.

157 Ko JM, Rodriguez HP, Fairchild DG, Rodday AC, Safran DG. Paying for enhanced services: Comparing patients' experiences in a concierge and general medicine practice. *Patient.* 2009;2:95-103.

158 Schillinger D, Bindman A, Wang F, Stewart A, Piette J. Functional health literacy and the quality of physician-patient communication among diabetes patients. *Patient Educ Couns.* 2004;52:315-323.

159 Castro CM, Wilson C, Wang F, Schillinger D. Babel babble: physicians' use of unclarified medical jargon with patients. *Am J Health Behav.* 2007;31(Suppl 1):S85-S95.

160 Schillinger D, Piette J, Grumbach K, et al. Closing the loop: physician communication with diabetic patients who have low health literacy. *Arch Intern Med.* 2003;163:83-90.

161 Sleath B, Roter D, Chewning B, Svarstad B. Asking questions about medication: analysis of physician-patient interactions and physician perceptions. *Med Care.* 1999;37:1169-1173.

162 Sleath B, Tulsky JA, Peck BM, Thorpe J. Provider-patient communication about antidepressants among veterans with mental health conditions. *Am J Geriatr Pharmacother.* 2007;5:9-17.

163 Young HN, Bell RA, Epstein RM, Feldman MD, Kravitz RL. Types of information physicians provide when prescribing antidepressants. *J Gen Intern Med.* 2006;21:1172-1177.

164 Sudore RL, Schillinger D. Interventions to improve care for patients with limited health literacy. *J Clin Outcomes Manag.* 2009;16:20-29.

165 DeWalt DA. Low health literacy: epidemiology and interventions. *N C Med J.* 2007;68:327-330.

166 Edwards M, Davies M, Edwards A. What are the external influences on information exchange and shared decision-making in healthcare consultations: a meta-synthesis of the literature. *Patient Educ Couns.* 2009;75:37-52.

167 Joosten EA, DeFuentes-Merillas L, de Weert GH, Sensky T, van der Staak CP, de Jong CA. Systematic review of the effects of shared decision-making on patient satisfaction, treatment adherence and health status. *Psychother Psychosom.* 2008;77:219-226.

168 Tanis M. Health-related on-line forums: what's the big attraction? *J Health Commun.* 2008;13:698-714.

169 van Roosmalen MS, Stalmeier PF, Verhoef LC, et al. Randomized trial of a shared decision-making intervention consisting of trade-offs and individualized treatment information for BRCA1/2 mutation carriers. *J Clin Oncol.* 2004;22:3293-3301.

170 Ludman E, Katon W, Bush T, et al. Behavioural factors associated with symptom outcomes in a primary care-based depression prevention intervention trial. *Psychol Med.* 2003;33:1061-1070.

171 Joosten EA, de Jong CA, de Weert-van Oene GH, Sensky T, van der Staak CP. Shared decision-making reduces drug use and psychiatric severity in substance-dependent patients. *Psychother Psychosom.* 2009;78:245-253.

172 Nose M, Barbui C, Gray R, Tansella M. Clinical interventions for treatment non-adherence in psychosis: meta-analysis. *Br J Psychiatry.* 2003;183:197-206.

173 Braddock CH 3rd, Edwards KA, Hasenberg NM, Laidley TL, Levinson W. Informed decision making in outpatient practice: time to get back to basics. *JAMA.* 1999;282:2313-2320.

174 Street RL Jr, Gordon HS, Ward MM, Krupat E, Kravitz RL. Patient participation in medical consultations: why some patients are more involved than others. *Med Care.* 2005;43:960-969.

175 Martins RK, McNeil DW. Review of motivational interviewing in promoting health behaviors. *Clinical Psychol Rev.* 2009;29:283-293.

176 Prochaska JO, DiClemente CC. Stages of change in the modification of problem behaviors. *Prog Behav Modif.* 1992;28:183-218.

177 Miller WR, Rollnick S. *Motivational Interviewing: Prepapring People to Change Addictive Behaviors*. New York, NY: Guilford Press; 1991.

178 Resnicow K, Jackson A, Wang T, et al. A motivational interviewing intervention to increase fruit and vegetable intake through Black churches: results of the Eat for Life trial. *Am J Public Health*. 2001;91:1686-1693.

179 Ogedegbe G, Chaplin W, Schoenthaler A, et al. A practice-based trial of motivational interviewing and adherence in hypertensive African Americans. *Am J Hypertens*. 2008;21:1137-1143.

180 Kemp R, Kirov G, Everitt B, Hayward P, David A. Randomised controlled trial of compliance therapy. 18-month follow-up. *Br J Psychiatry*. 1998;172:413-419.

181 Bellack AS, Bennett ME, Gearon JS, Brown CH, Yang Y. A randomized clinical trial of a new behavioral treatment for drug abuse in people with severe and persistent mental illness. *Arch Gen Psychiatry*. 2006;63:426-432.

182 West DS, DiLillo V, Bursac Z, Gore SA, Greene PG. Motivational interviewing improves weight loss in women with type 2 diabetes. *Diabetes Care*. 2007;30:1081-1087.

183 Bozovich M, Rubino CM, Edmunds J. Effect of a clinical pharmacist-managed lipid clinic on achieving National Cholesterol Education Program low-density lipoprotein goals. *Pharmacotherapy*. 2000;20:1375-1383.

184 Lee JK, Grace KA, Taylor AJ. Effect of a pharmacy care program on medication adherence and persistence, blood pressure, and low-density lipoprotein cholesterol: a randomized controlled trial. *JAMA*. 2006;296:2563-2571.

185 Nietert PJ, Tilley BC, Zhao W, et al. Two pharmacy interventions to improve refill persistence for chronic disease medications: a randomized, controlled trial. *Med Care*. 2009;47:32-40.

186 Raebel MA, Charles J, Dugan J, et al. Randomized trial to improve prescribing safety in ambulatory elderly patients. *J Am Geriatr Soc*. 2007;55:977-985.

187 Steele AW, Eisert S, Witter J, et al. The effect of automated alerts on provider ordering behavior in an outpatient setting. *PLoS Med*. 2005;2:e255.

188 Piette JD, Weinberger M, Kraemer FB, McPhee SJ. Impact of automated calls with nurse follow-up on diabetes treatment outcomes in a Department of Veterans Affairs Health Care System: a randomized controlled trial. *Diabetes Care*. 2001;24:202-208.

189 Piette JD, Weinberger M, McPhee SJ. The effect of automated calls with telephone nurse follow-up on patient-centered outcomes of diabetes care: a randomized controlled trial. *Med Care*. 2000;38:218-230.

190 Friedman RH, Kazis LE, Jette A, et al. A telecommunications system for monitoring and counseling patients with hypertension. Impact on medication adherence and blood pressure control. *Am J Hypertens*. 1996;9:285-292.

191 Russel M. *Behavioral Counseling in Medicine: Strategies for Modifying At-risk Behavior*. New York, NY: Oxford University Press; 1986.

192 Taylor CB, Miller NH. The behavioral approach. In: Wenger NK, Weinstein HK, ed. *Rehabiliation of the Coronary Patient*. New York, NY: Churchill Livingstone; 1992:461-471.

193 Heyscue BE, Levin GM, Merrick JP. Compliance with depot antipsychotic medication by patients attending outpatient clinics. *Psychiatr Serv*. 1998;49:1232-1234.

194 Patton K, Meyers J, Lewis BE. Enhancement of compliance among patients with hypertension. *Am J Manag Care*. 1997;3:1693-1698.

195 Berkman LF. Assessing the physical health effects of social networks and social support. *Annu Rev Public Health*. 1984;5:413-432.

196 Cohen S. Social relationships and health. *Am Psychol*. 2004;59:676-684.

197 DiMatteo MR. Social support and patient adherence to medical treatment: A meta-analysis. *Health Psychology*. 2004;23:207-218.

198 McCann BS, Retzlaff BM, Dowdy AA, Walden CE, Knopp RH. Promoting adherence to low-fat, low-cholesterol diets: Review and recommendations. *J Am Diet Assoc*. 1990;90:1408-1414.

199 Bovbjerg VE, McCann BS, Brief DJ, et al. Spouse support and long-term adherence to lipid-lowering diets. *Am J Epidemiol.* 1995;141:451-460.

200 Catz SL, Kelly JA, Bogart LM, Benotsch EG, McAuliffe TL. Patterns, correlates, and barriers to medication adherence among persons prescribed new treatments for HIV disease. *Health Psychol.* 2000;19:124-133.

201 Sherbourne CD, Hays RD, Ordway L, DiMatteo MR, Kravitz RL. Antecedents of adherence to medical recommendations: results from the Medical Outcomes Study. *J Behav Med.* 1992;15:447-468.

202 Molassiotis A, Nahas-Lopez V, Chung WY, Lam SW, Li CK, Lau TF. Factors associated with adherence to antiretroviral medication in HIV-infected patients. *Int J STD AIDS.* 2002;13:301-310.

203 Voils C, Steinhauser K, McCant F, Oddone E, Bosworth H. Understanding adherence to blood pressure-lowering regimens: A qualitative study of facilitators and barriers. In: *Health Services Research & Development National Meeting.* Baltimore; 2005.

204 Kopjar B, Sales AE, Pineros SL, Sun H, Li YF, Hedeen AN. Adherence with statin therapy in secondary prevention of coronary heart disease in veterans administration male population. *Am J Cardiol.* 2003;92:1106-1108.

205 Pratt J, Jones JJ. Noncompliance with therapy: an ongoing problem in treating hypertension. *Prim Cardiol.* 1995;21:34-38.

206 Urquhart J. Correlates of variable patient compliance in drug trials: relevance in the new health care environment. *Adv Drug Res.* 1995;26:237-257.

207 Sivarajan ES, Newton KM, Almes MJ, Kempf TM, Mansfield LW, Bruce RA. Limited effects of outpatient teaching and counseling after myocardial infarction: a controlled study. *Heart Lung.* 1983;12:65-73.

208 Haynes R, Sackett DL, Gibson ES, Taylor DW, Hackett BC, Roberts RS, Johnson AL. Improvement of medication compliance in uncontrolled hypertension. *Lancet.* 1976;1:1265-1268.

209 Bailey WC, Richards JM Jr, Brooks CM, Soong SJ, Windsor RA, Manzella BA. A randomized trial to improve self-management practices of adults with asthma. *Arch Intern Med.* 1990;150:1664-1668.

210 Ciechanowski PS, Katon WJ, Russo JE, Walker EA. The patient-provider relationship: attachment theory and adherence to treatment in diabetes. *Am J Psychiatry.* 2001;158:29-35.

211 Alexander SC, Sleath B, Golin CE, Kalinowski CT. Patient-Provider communication. In: Bosworth HB, Oddone EZ, Weinberger M, ed. *Patient treatment adherence: Concepts, interventions, and measurement.* Mahwah, NJ: Lawrence Erlbaum Associates; 2006.

212 Bender BG. Overcoming barriers to nonadherence in asthma treatment. *J Allergy Clin Immunol.* 2002;109:S554-S559.

213 Horne R. Patients' beliefs about treatment: the hidden determinant of treatment outcome? *J Psychosom Res.* 1999;47:491-495.

214 Yusuf S, Sleight P, Pogue J, Bosch J, Davies R, Dagenais G. Effects of an angiotensin-converting-enzyme inhibitor, ramipril, on cardiovascular events in high-risk patients. The Heart Outcomes Prevention Evaluation Study Investigators. *N Engl J Med.* 2000;342:145-153.